# *Acquired Hearing Loss*

## PSYCHOLOGICAL AND PSYCHOSOCIAL IMPLICATIONS

# *Acquired Hearing Loss*

## PSYCHOLOGICAL AND PSYCHOSOCIAL IMPLICATIONS

ALAN J. THOMAS

*Department of Applied Social Studies*
*Polytechnic of North London*
*London, United Kingdom*

1984

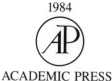

ACADEMIC PRESS

*(Harcourt Brace Jovanovich, Publishers)*

London   Orlando   San Diego   New York
Toronto   Montreal   Sydney   Tokyo

ACADEMIC PRESS INC (LONDON) LTD
24-28 Oval Road,
London NW1 7DX


*United States Edition published by*
ACADEMIC PRESS, INC.
Orlando, Florida 32887


Library of Congress Cataloging in Publication Data

Thomas, Alan J.
  Acquired hearing loss.

  Bibliography: p.
  Includes index.
  1. Deafness--Psychological aspects.  I. Title.
HV2395.T47  1984        362.4'23'019        84-12363
ISBN 0-12-687920-6 (alk. paper)


PRINTED IN THE UNITED STATES OF AMERICA

84 85 86 87      9 8 7 6 5 4 3 2 1

# *Foreword*

In the four decades since World War II, a number of important studies have been made of the psychological and psychosocial consequences of prelingual hearing loss. Despite the fact that individuals with acquired, postlingual hearing loss are at least 100 times more common, they have hitherto been neglected. Alan Thomas's monograph constitutes an important first step in remedying this neglect.

The differences between the two groups are worth considering. The prelingual group in many ways constitutes a distinct subset of the population, differing markedly in their means of communication, and so has attracted the interest of psychologists and linguists for theoretical as well as practical reasons. Those with hearing loss acquired after development of language are merely the general population with a blunted auditory input, a view supported by the findings of the two studies reported in this book. It is to be expected, therefore, that the changes to be found will be far more subtle.

What is surprising is the degree of psychological change found in certain of the present groups—from 18–19% in the basic study groups to 57% in one subset—compared with 5% in a normally hearing control group. The reasons for this aspect of handicap are examined and discussed at considerable length, with much detail provided of other aspects of handicap experienced by these hearing-impaired individuals.

The approach to impairment–disability–handicap used in this publication follows Wood's system—now adopted by the World Health Organization and discussed in some detail by Duckworth (1983). This in itself constitutes an important basis for any real consideration of the consequences of ear damage on the individual concerned, and it seems pertinent to quote Alan

Thomas's words from the concluding section of the book: "The expectation that knowledge about the disorder, impairment, and disability domains of auditory dysfunction would lead to a better understanding of the nature of hearing impairment has not been fulfilled. Moreover, it does not seem likely that current research in the first three domains will yield very much information which could be put to practical use for some time to come."

It is important, however, to state that in his studies, Dr. Thomas has highlighted many important ways in which the problems of hearing handicap can be approached, and I expect this book to provide the starting point for many studies.

S. D. G. STEPHENS
*Royal National Throat, Nose, and Ear Hospital*
*London, United Kingdom*

# *Preface*

One-sixth of the adult population of Britain acquires a significant hearing loss in adult life. Very little is known about the disorder or about the effect that it has on people's lives. During recent years, however, a certain amount of research on acquired hearing loss has been initiated. The purpose of this book is to fill a gap in this research by describing what I believe to be the first-ever systematic investigation into the psychological and psychosocial effects of acquired hearing loss in adults of working age. In particular, this book examines the effect of hearing loss on mental health and psychological well-being, work, family, and social life. It then relates findings in these areas to audiological variables such as onset, type and degree of hearing loss, speech comprehension, and the amount of benefit obtained from a hearing aid. Implications for rehabilitation are also considered. Indeed, given that the book focusses on people who have owned a hearing aid for at least a year, it can also be viewed as an evaluation of existing rehabilitation services.

It is hoped that the book will prove useful for those whose professional work brings them into contact with the hearing impaired, and for social scientists, researchers, and members of the caring professions who want to know more about what it means to live with a communication disability.

The research programme described in the book was carried out in the Department of Applied Social Studies at the Polytechnic of North London. It was funded mainly by the Medical Research Council and partly by the Polytechnic of North London through the allocation of research posts. Much of the initial work was supported by a fellowship funded by the Royal National Institute for the Deaf. I gratefully acknowledge Dr. Katia

Gilhome Herbst's collaboration in setting up the research programme and in codirecting the first of the two studies that make up the programme.

I would like to thank Dr. S. D. G. Stephens, Consultant in Audiological Medicine at the Royal National Throat, Nose, and Ear Hospital, London, and Professor C. I. Howarth, Department of Psychology, University of Nottingham, for their very helpful comments on various drafts and sections of the book and also Mr. M. Martin, OBE, of the Royal National Institute for the Deaf, for his invaluable technical advice.

I gratefully acknowledge the contribution of those appointed to the research programme for varying periods of time: Liz Dawtrey, Margaret Harris, Sue Humphries, Dr. Margaret Lamont, Jim Ring, and Janet Stevenson. I would also like to thank erstwhile colleagues at the Polytechnic of North London for their support: Dr. Paul Corrigan, Dr. Bob Gilchrist, John Hall, Mike Hayes, Gill Madge, Terence Miller, Jean Snelling, and Arthur Verney. I am especially indebted to Maureen Fedarb for typing numerous drafts of the manuscript.

The following organisations supported the research programme in various ways: the Royal National Institute for the Deaf, the British Association of the Hard-of-Hearing, the City Literary Institute Centre for the Deaf, the Royal National Throat, Nose, and Ear Hospital, University College Hospital, the Royal Northern Hospital, Charing Cross Hospital, Hillingdon Hospital, The London Hospital, Guys Hospital, St. Thomas's Hospital, and St. Mary Abbotts Hospital, all in London.

*ALAN J. THOMAS**

*Present address: Department of Education Studies, Darwin Institute of Technology, Darwin, Australia.

# Contents

## Part III: The Second Study:
## Severe Sensorineural Hearing Loss

## Chapter 5: Methodology and Audiological Characteristics

## Chapter 6: Psychological and Psychosocial Effects

## Chapter 7: Overview and Implications for Rehabilitation

*Written with Margaret Lamont and Margaret Harris.

# PART ONE

*Background*

# CHAPTER ONE

# *Introduction*

## I. PRELIMINARY CONSIDERATIONS

The terms *hearing impairment* and *the hearing impaired* are gradually replacing those of *deafness* and *the deaf*, respectively, mainly because of the negative connotations associated with the latter terms. In a similar vein, the term *hearing loss* now tends to be used instead of *acquired* or *adventitious deafness*. The terminology used in this book will be, as far as possible, in keeping with these changes.

The consequences of hearing impairment differ greatly depending on age of onset, type of impairment, severity of hearing loss, and so on. The most important and fundamental distinction is between prelingual and postlingual hearing impairment. Prelingual hearing impairment will almost certainly interfere with the acquisition of speech and language. Educational achievement is affected to such an extent that children leaving schools for the hearing impaired at the age of 16 are, on average, 8 years behind their hearing peers; speech production is so affected as to make their speech unintelligible to all but closest acquaintances (DES, 1963; Denmark, 1973; Conrad, 1977; Denmark *et al.*, 1979). It is not surprising, therefore, that a large section of the prelingually hearing-impaired population forms a unique subculture whose separate identity is reinforced by the extensive use of sign language as a means of communication. In fact, about 90% of marriages involving the prelingually hearing impaired are with similarly affected partners (Schein and Delk, 1975). Research into the psychological and educational consequences of prelingual hearing impairment has expanded considerably over the last 20 years or so, and a number of general texts have appeared (Levine, 1960; Myklebust, 1964; Furth, 1966; Mindel and Vernon, 1971; Frisina, 1976; Conrad, 1979).

When onset of hearing loss occurs after the normal acquisition of language and speech, the effects are obviously quite different. In spite of this, a number of writers have not fully grasped the distinction, perhaps because "deafness" and "hearing impairment" are used as blanket terms. Remmers and Wright (1960) and Cattell *et al.* (1970), for example, have attempted to obtain norms for the deaf for an adjustment inventory and for a personality questionnaire, respectively, without indicating to what type of deafness the norms refer. A definition of hearing impairment in a book on the psychology of handicap also fails to make the distinction (Shakespeare, 1975).

> Hearing impairment includes deafness and partial hearing. Again the degree varies, the impairment may be almost complete, the person may be able to hear some sounds but not others or be generally a little hard-of-hearing [p. 136].

Even researchers who take hearing loss as their starting point have sometimes failed to grasp the distinction. Knapp (1948) and Mahapatra (1974a,b) quote studies of prelingually hearing-impaired adults as analogous to their own studies of adults with acquired hearing loss. A psychiatrist who specialises in hearing impairment has even felt it necessary to make the distinction explicit in a medical journal (Denmark, 1969).

> Those suffering from a profound prelingual deafness suffer a sensory deficit; those deafened in adult life suffer a sensory deprivation. The problems of the one are developmental, of the other traumatic. They cannot be equated [p. 965].

Evidence from a number of sources attests to the paucity of research on the psychological and psychosocial effects of acquired hearing loss. A monograph supplement on hearing loss in the *British Journal of Audiology* does not cite one reference in a chapter entitled "Psychosocial Effects" (Markides, 1977). The "Rawson Report" (DHSS, 1973), concerned with the promotion of research into hearing loss in general, specifically referred to the dearth of research into social and psychological implications, as also did Cooper in a review of the relationship between hearing impairment and psychiatric illness (Cooper, 1976).

A brief consideration of possible effects of hearing loss underlines the need for systematic research. By disrupting conversation, hearing loss might be expected to impose a strain on interpersonal relationships. Subsequent withdrawal from social contact might result in isolation and loneliness. [Those who rely heavily on contact with the hearing-impaired person (e.g., family members) may also suffer from the effects of impaired communication.] Little solace may be gained from association with "the own" (Goffman, 1963), who suffer from the same handicap, the point being that conversation can become well-nigh impossible between hearing-impaired persons. It is also popularly believed, though little documented, that misunderstandings and not knowing what people are saying result in a heightened state of suspiciousness. Loss of contact with background sounds, which normally serve to keep us in constant touch with the everyday world, might have a disorienting effect. Such considerations lead one to expect that the consequences of hearing loss for personal well-being, and for social, family, and work life, will be profound.

It is true, of course, that much can be done to remedy hearing loss. Certain types of hearing loss can be treated surgically or medically. The majority who suffer from an irreversible type of hearing loss (usually sensorineural) may benefit from wearing a hearing aid. However, many hearing-impaired people, for a variety of reasons, obtain relatively little benefit from the use of a hearing aid and are usually encouraged to develop lip-reading skills. Contrary to popular belief, however, few sounds can be "read," and those that can are mostly vowels, which contribute little to meaning—try leaving vowels out of a sentence as opposed to consonants. While a few hearing-impaired individuals are undeniably good lip-readers, the vast majority make little if any progress, even after prolonged attendance at lip-reading classes (Skamris, 1974; McCormick, 1979a; Stephens, 1979a; Summerfield, 1983). In recent years, the new specialisms of audiological medicine and hearing therapy have appeared. Given the large residual disability likely to remain after the acquisition of a hearing aid, an important part of the work of these professionals is to help the impaired person to live with his or her hearing loss. A better developed understanding of the psychological and psychosocial consequences of hearing loss would seem to be essential for this task.

A focus on the psychological and psychosocial aspects of hearing loss reflects developments in the study of disability in general. In her major study of handicapped people in Great Britain, Harris (1971) distinguishes between impairment, disability, and handicap, giving the term *handicap* a specific meaning as distinct from the general one, which is more usually employed. For Harris, *impairment* means "lacking part or all of a limb, or having a defective limb, organ, or mechanism of the body." *Disablement* is defined as "the loss or reduction of functional ability," and *handicap* as "the disadvantage or restriction of activity caused by the disability." Harris gives the following hypothetical example of the relationship between disability and handicap (Harris, 1971).

> A man has had a leg amputated. Therefore he is impaired, and since he would have a reduction in his locomotor ability, he is disabled. If, however, he has a satisfactory prothesis, a sedentary job, a car adjusted to hand controls and leisure activities which are not too active, he might well not be restricted in activity and therefore not handicapped [p. 2].

The problem with this example is that it confines itself to practical aspects of handicap and neglects the equally important effect of disability on psychological well-being and on the *quality* of social, family, and work life. Davis (1983) has adapted Harris's schema and expressed it in terms of auditory dysfunction (Table 1.1). The main difference is that Davis distinguishes between locus of impairment, which he terms *disorder,* and abnormal function, which he terms *impairment.* He also goes much further than Harris in recognizing the importance of psychological and psychosocial factors in the handicap domain.

Shakespeare (1975), adopting a rather different approach, makes a clear distinction between personal and practical adjustment to disability. Her criteria for successful practical adjustment include having somewhere to live, being able to look after oneself, being able to keep out of trouble, and not depending too much on social agencies. In the area of personal adjustment she stresses the importance of "not behaving in a bizarre fashion or socially inappropriate manner." She also stresses the need to maintain adequate personal relationships in order "to avoid extensive loneliness and to avoid rejection through being unaware of other people's reactions; not interrupting or monopolising conversations or addressing strangers in a familiar manner . . . being able to contribute to friendship as well as receiving." Shakespeare's concern is with physically disabled people who develop inappropriate social styles in reaction to their disability. For the hearing impaired, such maladaptive behaviour may occur irrespective of genuine attempts to interact with others in a socially acceptable manner.

TABLE 1.1

Domains of Auditory Dysfunction[a]

| | Disorder | Impairment | Disability | Handicap |
|---|---|---|---|---|
| Definition | Pathology of the hearing organ | Abnormal function of the auditory system | Reduced abilities of the individual | Need for extra effort, Reduced independence |
| Area affected | Middle ear<br>Inner ear<br>Hair cells<br>Auditory nerve<br>Brainstem<br>Auditory cortex | Auditory sensitivity<br>Auditory discrimination<br>Auditory localisation<br>Temporal processing<br>Binaural integration<br>Tinnitus | Speech perception, Environmental awareness, Orientation | Grade of employment<br>Scope of employment<br>Remuneration<br>Personal relationships<br>Social integration<br>Anxiety, embarrassment |
| Appropriate remedial action | Medical and surgical treatment | Environmental and personal aids to hearing | | Counselling and special provisions |

[a]From Davis (1983).

Monopolising conversation, for example, may represent a genuine attempt to minimise the likelihood both of the embarrassment which arises from the need for constant repetition and of the social blunders caused by misunderstandings. The need to stand close to others in order to hear better can also be mistaken for overfamiliarity.

Other writers have also stressed the attention which should be given to psychological and psychosocial factors. Brattgard (1974) argues that adequate rehabilitation of the physically disabled population is impossible unless social and psychological factors are taken into account because "a disabled person runs the risk of isolation in the community and segregation from other people . . . if he lacks stimulating contacts with other human beings." McDaniel (1976) suggests that the social isolation experienced by the physically disabled, which results from interference with communication and mobility, may produce emotional distress in a manner similar to that which has been demonstrated for sensory isolation. He argues that "social isolation would not easily be overcome for those individuals who are confined to bed, home, hospitals, or other institutions for extended periods of time," mainly because the sufferers may be deprived of normal patterns of human interaction. McDaniel's views concern physical disability but are also relevant to hearing impairment because he believes it is necessary to turn to isolation resulting from "permanent, partial, or total loss of a receptor system" in order to illustrate the damaging effects of social isolation.

The twofold aim of this book is to attempt to (a) quantify and (b) gain insights into the psychological and psychosocial handicap which remains after a hearing aid has been prescribed and used (or not used) for a minimum of 1 year by adults of working age. Part I of the book (Chapters 1 and 2) serves as a background to the research programme which forms the bulk of the book. The two studies which comprise the research programme are described in Parts II and III, respectively. The following summary should enable the reader to obtain a grasp of the overall scope of the programme:

## FIRST STUDY

Sample based on owners of National Health Service hearing aids irrespective of degree or type of hearing loss

$N = 211$ adults of employment age

Speech discrimination ability for single words presented aurally

Standardised measure of psychological disturbance

Interview schedule containing structured items on employment, social and family life, suspiciousness, and personal well-being, all controlled on general population studies.

Questions about hearing-aid usage, use of services, and adjustment to hearing loss

## SECOND STUDY

Sample based on owners of National Health Service hearing aids with sensorineural hearing loss ranging from moderately severe to total

$N = 88$ adults of employment age

Speech tests for single words as in the First Study and for words presented audiovisually

Standardised measure of hearing handicap as perceived by the individual

Detailed checklist of problems likely to be encountered at work

Standardised personality inventory

Standardised measure of psychological disturbance as in the First Study

Structured items concerning onset of hearing loss and use of hearing aid

## Family Study

Sample: family members and close friends of 27 respondents who took part in the second study

Method: open-ended interviews conducted in respondents' homes

The final chapter reviews the major findings from both studies and considers the implications for rehabilitation.

## II. THE NATURE OF HEARING LOSS

### A. Hearing

The ear is usually thought of as divided into three parts: outer, middle, and inner (Fig. 1.1). The outer ear consists of the auricle, which is the visible part of the ear, and the external auditory canal. The external auditory canal conducts airborne sound waves to the tympanic membrane (ear

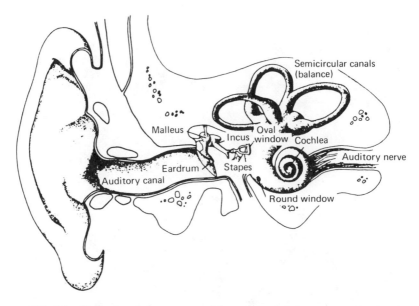

FIG. 1.1. Illustration of the structure of the peripheral auditory system showing the outer, middle, and inner ear. Adapted from *Human Information Processing* by Lindsey and Norman (1972) by permission of the authors.

drum), which separates the outer ear from the middle ear. Sound waves entering the ear cause the tympanic membrane to vibrate. The middle ear is an air-filled cavity which contains a series of three small bones, or ossicles: the hammer (*malleus*), anvil (*incus*), and stirrup (*stapes*). Vibration of the tympanic membrane causes these three bones to vibrate in turn. Movement of the stapes at the oval window, which marks the boundary between the middle and inner ear, causes pressure waves to travel through the peri-lymph and endolymph fluids of the inner ear. Hence, sound is conducted in turn by air, bone, and fluid. Variations in fluid pressure of the inner ear stimulate sensory hair cells located in the cochlea. It is in the cochlea that the first stage of acoustical analysis occurs before information is transmit-ted via the auditory (cochlear) nerve to the higher auditory centres of the temporal lobe of the brain. While this description of the mechanism is highly simplified, it is sufficient for an understanding of the different types of hearing loss which will now be described.

## B. Conductive Hearing Loss

The term *conductive hearing loss* is usually applied to hearing loss which arises from a middle ear disease. The most common form of conductive hearing loss, however, is caused by the accumulation of wax in the outer ear. The presence of a foreign body will also interfere with air conduction of sound. In either case, removal is almost always straightforward. An infection of the outer ear (*otitis externa*) can also cause a significant hearing loss, although a return to normal hearing can be expected if and when the condition clears or is cleared.

*Acute otitis media* and *otosclerosis* are the diseases usually associated with conductive hearing loss in the middle ear. Acute otitis media is the name given to infections which result in the inflammation of the mucous membranes of the middle ear. The condition may cause fluid to accumulate in the normally air-filled, middle ear cavity (*seromucous otitis media,* or "glue ear.") It is very common in early childhood; 75% of cases occur in children under 10 years of age (MRC, 1957). If the condition does not clear, certain drainage procedures may be carried out. Acute otitis media may become chronic as a result of perforation of the tympanic membrane, from further secondary infection, or through fibrosis of the middle ear. Otosclerosis is a disease in which the final bone in the ossicular chain, the stapes, gradually becomes firmly fixed in the oval window, thus preventing effective transmission of vibrations from the other bones in the ossicular chain to the fluid of the inner ear. The disease, which is basically genetic, though of unknown cause, can be treated surgically by a stapedectomy, which may restore normal or near-normal bone conduction.

A conductive hearing loss is not usually regarded as serious because it can usually be treated medically or surgically. Moreover, a hearing aid is well suited to a conductive hearing loss. If the inner ear is normal, the only imperfections in the sound input should be attributable to the aid itself. However, the effects of conductive hearing loss are not necessarily straightforward. Peterson and Gross (1972) point out that "conductive impairment arising from more than one part of the conductive apparatus may make the system more nonlinear in its action and thus increase the distortion of the acoustic waveforms that reach the sense organ . . . any nonlinear distortion will not only not be corrected, but is likely to become worse when the input signal is increased in order to deliver more acoustic energy to the same organ.''

The endolymph and perilymph fluids of the inner ear are also concerned with conduction of sound. The most common disorder associated with these fluids, *Ménière's disorder,* causes fluctuations in hearing ability which may include recovery of normal hearing for long periods. The disorder can result in an eventual sensorineural loss, however, as the excessive pressure caused by the hydrops increasingly affects the cochlea. The cause of Ménière's disorder is unknown, although a number of theories have been postulated including one that it is psychosomatic in origin (e.g., Hinchcliffe, 1967; Czubalski *et al.,* 1976).

## C. Sensorineural Hearing Loss

*Sensorineural hearing loss* is also referred to as inner ear, perceptive, or ''nerve'' hearing loss. Sensory hearing loss originates in the inner ear, while neural hearing loss is caused by lesions in the auditory nerve which transmits information from the inner ear to the brain. For present purposes, the blanket term will be adhered to simply because both sensory and neural losses are almost without exception permanent and irreversible. Incidentally, the vast majority of such losses is predominantly sensory or cochlear.

The most common cause of sensorineural hearing loss is *presbyacusis,* or ''old-age deafness.'' There is some evidence that presbyacusis is not simply a degenerative disease, based on the finding that elderly people in primitive societies have better hearing than those in modern industrial societies (Rosen *et al.,* 1962). Factors such as exposure to excessive noise, heredity, survival of the less healthy, experiences of ototoxic drugs, stress, high blood pressure, and diet may all contribute to the difference between the two types of societies. In fact, a comparison of the hearing levels associated with age in the Mabaan tribe and in North Americans at the Wisconsin State Fair in 1954 seems to demonstrate that degenerative changes play little part in the onset of ''old-age deafness'' in modern societies (Glorig *et al.,* 1957). More recently, Stephens (1979b) has queried the existence of presbyacusis as a degenerative disease in that many of its forms can be explained in terms of other aetiological factors such as those described above.

Pliny and Bacon are among a number of well-known writers who have commented on loss of hearing due to noise. Ballantyne (1977) notes that in 1831, Fosbroke reported deafness in blacksmiths, and Barr (1886) first described *boilermakers' deafness,* a term still used today. Explosions, blasts, and sudden noises can cause immediate hearing loss which may be temporary or permanent. Hearing loss caused by long-term exposure to industrial (or similar) noise is always permanent. The seriousness of this type of hearing loss derives from its almost imperceptible onset and insidious progress, which may occur over many years. Resistance to cumbersome protective devices is understandable, especially given the adverse effect they have on social discourse. The popular belief that exposure to loud music causes hearing loss has not been substantiated.

The onset of sensorineural hearing loss in childhood, adolescence, or later may be associated with hereditary factors acting on the hearing mechanism alone or in conjunction with other abnormalities. Sensorineural hearing loss can also be induced by taking certain drugs, which usually gain access to the inner ear via the bloodstream. Quinine and nicotine are among a number of drugs which have been associated with hearing loss. Certain antibiotics have also been shown to cause hearing loss, the most well-known being streptomycin, used to treat tuberculosis. Viral and bacterial infections can also cause hearing loss, usually in children. Maternal rubella in the first 3 months of pregnancy, for example, is known to be associated with congenital deafness. Mumps and measles are among other infections which may result in a sensorineural hearing loss.

## D. Other Factors

There are a number of complications or side effects associated with hearing loss. Tinnitus, recruitment, and vertigo are the most common. Tinnitus (rather ironically) is a condition in which noises or ringing in the head or ears occurs. While it is most commonly associated with sensorineural hearing loss, it can accompany conductive loss and normal hearing. *Subjective* tinnitus is perceived by the sufferer alone, and there is almost always no known physiological correlate. *Objective* tinnitus, a much rarer condition, can be "heard" by an observer and usually explained in physiological terms. The phenomenon of recruitment, commonly associated with hearing loss, means that a slight increase in sound above threshold results in a disproportionate increase in the sensation of sound. Hence, the dynamic range for hearing may be reduced. In some cases, fairly loud sounds which are quite acceptable to the normally hearing may cause discomfort or even pain to those with hearing impairment.

Central hearing impairment is concerned with disorders which occur beyond the auditory nerve, that is, between the brainstem and the cerebral cortex. Though not directly relevant, it is worth mentioning briefly. The nature of the disorder may be physiological or psychological in origin. Actual brain damage, caused by, for example, thrombosis, tumour, meningitis, or senility, may also result in hearing loss. Psychogenic deafness has been known to result from extremely stressful life events, especially wartime ones. Such hearing loss is usually (but not always) of short duration. Psychotic conditions may also be accompanied by hearing loss. Whether forms of central hearing loss related to a known psychopathology are truly forms of deafness is open to question. Chaiklin and Ventry (1963), for example, have shown that adults suffering from psychogenic deafness constitute a problem category that is distinct from acquired hearing impairment, which is known to be organic in origin.

## E.  Prevalence of Hearing Loss

The first systematic attempt to estimate the prevalence of hearing impairment in Britain was undertaken by Wilkins, who in 1947 carried out a survey aimed at gauging the demand for hearing aids following the advent of the National Health Service (Wilkins, 1948). Self-estimates of hearing ability were obtained, respondents being asked to place themselves on the scale contained in Table 1.2. The table also gives the number found at each level of the scale. Wilkins's estimate for the prevalence within each age group was as follows:

| Age (years) | Percentage |
|-------------|------------|
| 25–44       | 1.6        |
| 45–64       | 4.7        |
| 65–74       | 12.2       |
| 75+         | 27.0       |

TABLE 1.2

Summary from Survey of the Prevalence of Deafness[a]

| Degree of Hearing Loss | N[b] |
|---|---|
| 1. Can hear all normal speech without an aid. | — |
| 2. The same as 1, but with one defective ear. | — |
| 3. Can hear speech at close range without an aid, but has difficulty in group conversation and in hearing in church or theatre. | 860,000 |
| 4. Has difficulty with normal speech but can hear loudly spoken speech. | 790,000 |
| 5. Has difficulty with loud speech but can hear amplified speech. | 70,000 |
| 6. Cannot hear speech at all but became deaf after normally learning speech. | 30,000 |
| 7. Deaf mutes, or became deaf early in life, and did not acquire speech normally. | 15,000 |

[a]From Wilkins, 1948, based on findings from a survey of the population of England, Scotland, and Wales.

[b]N, number of people in each category.

A United States study, based on the collection of audiometric data, found a prevalence rate of 1.6% for a loss between 41 and 55 decibels (dB), and 1.1% for a loss in excess of 55 dB, thus making a total prevalence rate of 2.7% (United States Department of Health, Education and Welfare, 1965).

With regard to the working age population (on which the studies described in this book are based), an audiometric study of a general practice in Kent found 5.8% of a sample of 2278 adults between 40 and 64 years of age to suffer a bilateral hearing loss in excess of 30 dB averaged across the frequencies of 500, 1000, and 2000 hertz (Hz) (D'Souza et al. 1975). MacAdam et al. (1981) reported a prevalence rate of 2% for the 16–44 age range and 7% for those between 45 and 64, based on the criterion of 35 dB unilateral hearing loss at 1000 Hz. The proportion with a bilateral hearing loss, however, was small: "Among the deaf, 18% were deaf in both ears," thus reducing the proportion far below that reported by D'Souza and his associates.

First phase results from the National Study of Hearing seem to demonstrate that prevalence is much higher than that suggested by earlier studies (Davis, 1983). Davis reports a prevalence rate of 17 ± 2.2%, ranging from 1% in young adults through 23% for those in their fifties to 74% for the over-seventies. These markedly higher rates can be explained in part by the criteria which Davis uses for classification as hearing impaired—a loss of 25 dB across the frequencies of 500, 1000, 2000, and 4000 Hz. Most earlier studies are based on 30dB and do not include the frequency of 4000 Hz, hearing for which is known to deteriorate at a much faster rate with increasing age and which many believe to be outside the frequency range important for the discrimination of speech. On the other hand, Haggard *et al.* (1981a) argue convincingly that the criteria used in the National Study of Hearing are better indicators of hearing impairment in real-life situations. Incidentally, Gilhome Herbst and Humphrey (1981), in a community study of the elderly (aged 70 and over), reported a prevalence rate of 60% based on a hearing loss of 35 dB averaged across the frequencies of 1000, 2000, and 4000 Hz.

## F. Measurement of Hearing Loss

### 1. *Pure Tone Audiometry*

The hearing thresholds for pure tones across a range of frequencies provide an individual profile of hearing ability known as the *pure tone audiogram*. The hearing threshold is measured in decibels on a logarithmic scale. The baseline of 0 dB is arbitrarily derived from the threshold of hearing of healthy young male conscripts. Frequencies are measured in cycles per second (cps) or hertz, two names for the same measure. Measurement of hearing ability is normally confined to the frequency range of 250–8000 Hz, which covers almost all speech sounds, although most speech is contained within the 500–4000 Hz frequency range.

As a rough guide to the measurement of sound intensity, a whisper at 3 ft is 30 dB above threshold, light traffic is around 50 dB, a conversational voice is 60 dB, a pneumatic drill is 90 dB or greater, and jet aircraft at takeoff is at least 125 dB. As might be expected, there is wide variation in noise tolerance. Some experience discomfort well below 120 dB, and almost all experience pain above 140 dB. With regard to frequency, the lowest note on the piano is 31 Hz, a foghorn has a frequency of about 100 Hz, middle C on the piano is at 256 Hz, the radio news pips are at 1000 Hz, and top C on the piano is at 4096 Hz. A bat squeak ranges between 8000 and 120,000 Hz. The range of frequencies audible to the human ear is roughly between about 20 and 20,000 Hz. Pure tones at specific frequencies are highly artificial and are rarely heard in everyday situations. Indeed, nearly all sounds are highly complex, with regard to both frequency and intensity.

In a typical testing situation, a person listens to pure tones, at varying frequencies and intensities, through headphones in a soundproofed or very quiet room. The intention of the test is to establish a hearing threshold for all or some of the frequencies between 250 and 8000 Hz. For research purposes, and often for policy decisions, it is common to take the mean or weighted mean of dB loss at a given number of frequencies covering the range for speech. The drawback to this procedure is that profiles which may have very different consequences for speech perception can have the same mean dB loss. Figure 1.2 contains three audiograms taken from one of the studies to be described in this book. They clearly illustrate that a single index of hearing loss can be highly misleading.

A variant of pure tone audiometry can be used to determine type of hearing loss. In this case, hearing ability for pure tones is measured by placing a vibrator on the mastoid bone behind the ear. This allows sound waves to be transmitted directly to the inner ear through the bones of the skull, thus bypassing any middle ear malfunction. Hearing by "bone conduction," as it is known, cannot be worse than for air conduction. If it is significantly better (i.e., a difference of 15 to 20 dB), then interference with the conduction of sound in the middle ear region can be inferred. A comparison of the bone and air audiogram profiles enables type of hearing loss to be determined as sensorineural, conductive, or "mixed" (i.e., the extent to which both conductive and sensorineural losses are present).

Pure tone audiometry has the advantage of being a standardised and highly reliable measure of hearing loss. Its main disadvantage is that it is normally carried out in an artificial, laboratory-type situation with stimuli which are almost never heard. It is for such reasons that attempts have been made to develop measures which reflect more closely the everyday effects of hearing loss, and these will now be described.

## 2. Speech Audiometry

Speech audiometry measures the ab lity to hear and understand speech. The rationale for the development of speech tests has been that pure tones

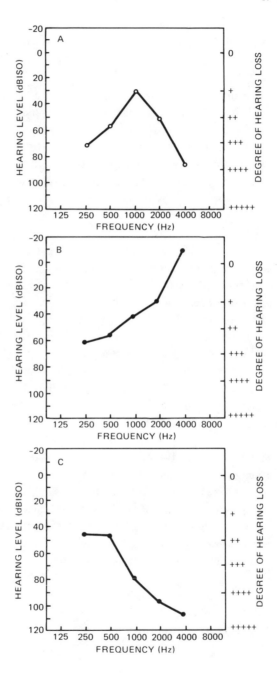

are rarely heard in everyday life, that people with similar audiometric profiles appear to differ widely in their ability to understand speech, and therefore that ability to discriminate speech will more accurately reflect the limitations imposed by hearing loss. Perhaps the best way to consider speech audiometry is firstly according to the nature of the speech material used, and secondly with reference to the conditions under which testing takes place.

Speech test material ranges from single nonsense syllables to prose passages, thus from a test of what a person can hear to one of what he can understand given contextual, linguistic, and other features of prose which aid comprehension. The most commonly used speech material consists of phonetically balanced, monosyllabic word lists which allow whole-word and phonemic scoring. Sentences used in speech testing have ranged from proverbs to ones in which a systematic effort has been made to control phonemic representation, frequency, and probability of word occurrence.

Speech may be presented in a variety of ways which will largely depend on the research or clinical question that the user is asking. For example, the intention may be to establish the level of output needed for the discrimination of speech, or speech may be presented at a normally acceptable level, with or without a hearing aid. Speech may be recorded or live, and output may be at any predetermined level (e.g., that of normal conversation). Material can be presented acoustically or audiovisually if the listener is to take advantage of gesture, facial movements, and lip patterns. A film or video sequence can allow situational clues to be utilised. In order to simulate everyday listening conditions, speech material may be presented against a background of white noise or conversational babble. Speech audiometry can also be used to assist in the differential diagnosis of sensory and neural hearing loss, as a guide to hearing aid selection, and in conjunction with pure tone audiometry to diagnose nonorganic hearing loss. It is used in conjunction with auditory training to diagnose difficulties in hearing for speech, and in order to evaluate the effect of training programmes.

FIG. 1.2.   Three hearing loss profiles showing that averaged dB losses can be misleading. Mean hearing loss for A, 58 dB; for B, 35 dB; for C, 74 dB. Degrees of hearing loss: 0, none; +, slight; + +, moderate; + + +, severe; + + + +, profound; + + + + +, total. (Examples are cases taken from the first study; ○ = left ear, ● = right ear.)

## 3. *Inventories of Handicap Due to Hearing Loss*

Noble (1978) summarises the drawbacks of speech tests:

> Speech tests that can be relied upon are so corseted in terms of content and style that they are freakish forms of speech as it is heard in the world at large. Conversely, those that try to emulate everyday conditions provide such widely variable results that no firm outcome emerges from their use . . . [and] no evidence is available to show that the speech test itself bears any relation to actual performance at listening or communicating in everyday conditions [p. 238].

As well as having little proven validity with regard to face-to-face communication, there is no evidence that speech tests are related to the ability to follow television and radio or to use the telephone. Neither can speech tests take into account the problems hearing-impaired individuals invariably meet in group conversations. Moreover, no account is taken of other aspects of hearing handicap, for example, difficulty in localisation of speech and nonspeech sounds, especially of warning signals. In order to obtain a measure of the overall handicapping effect of hearing loss, a number of self-report inventories have been constructed in which the individual rates his or her own hearing across a wide range of situations. By doing this, it is possible to overcome the problem of the artificiality of speech testing, which inevitably occurs in a laboratory-type testing situation. The individual's assessment of his or her own hearing disability will also take any effect due to personality, lifestyle, and particular environment into account.

Three such measures have been used fairly widely during the past 20 years or so. High *et al.* (1964) developed a Hearing Handicap Scale in the United States in order to provide an objective measure ''to complement the wealth of anecdotal material available.'' Similar indices have been developed in Denmark by Ewertsen and Birk Nielsen (1973) and in Britain by Noble and Atherley (1970). The Danish instrument, the Social Hearing Handicap Scale, has been translated into English. The American and Danish inventories are similar in nature, both constructed from observations of audiologists and otologists (ear surgeons) concerning the everyday effects of hearing loss. The type of question asked is illustrated in the following three items taken from High's Hearing Handicap Scale:

> Can you carry on a conversation with one other person when you are on a noisy street corner?

Can you hear warning signals, such as automobile horns, railway crossing bells, or emergency vehicle sirens?

When you are buying something in a store, do you easily understand the clerk?

In reviewing the two measures, Noble (1978) points out that a hearing handicap is defined by self-styled experts who have normal hearing and are "not much less ignorant than the population at large . . . when it comes to knowing the experienced world of the partially deaf person."

The Hearing Measure Scale (HMS) of Noble and Atherley (1970) was developed from interviews with people likely to have suffered from noise-induced hearing loss. They ranged from bus drivers, who would be expected to have the least degree of impairment, to boilermakers, who would be most likely to have a severe hearing loss. Analysis of the interviews led to the identification of seven areas of hearing disability. The title of each section is given below and is accompanied by an illustrative question.

Section 1   *Hearing for Speech*   Do you have difficulty hearing in group conversation at home?

Section 2   *Hearing for Nonspeech Sound*   Can you hear the clock ticking in the room?

Section 3   *Spatial Localisation*   Do you turn your head the wrong way when someone you can't see calls out to you?

Section 4   *Emotional Response*   Do you get bothered or upset if you are unable to follow a conversation?

Section 5   *Speech Distortion*   Do you find that announcers on tv/radio fail to speak clearly?

Section 6   *Tinnitus*   Do you get buzzing or ringing noises inside your head or ears?

Section 7   *Personal Opinion*   Does any difficulty in hearing restrict your social or personal life?

The HMS, which was originally developed for administration by interview, is now available in a form suitable for self-completion (Noble, 1979).

## G.  Aids and Appliances

### 1.  *Hearing Aids*

The time-honoured air-conduction hearing aid consists of a hand cupped behind the ear. Over the centuries various ear trumpets have been developed. Four nonelectrical hearing aids are still available under the National

Health Service. Electrical aids have existed since the end of the last century, although electronic advances made in the Second World War made possible the first truly portable, body-worn aid. It was pioneered mainly by the Medical Research Council to meet the demand following the founding of the National Health Service (NHS) in 1948. Over the next 25 years, bodyworn aids were the only ones issued by the NHS. The typical bodyworn aid consists of a microphone–amplifier unit in a box weighing a few ounces, which is usually clipped to clothing on the chest. Amplified output at the ear is conducted through an orifice in an individually made ear mould which fits into the exterior auditory canal. A bone-conduction hearing aid is similar except that amplified sound is transmitted through a vibrator pressed against the mastoid bone behind the ear, and thence directly to the inner ear, bypassing the defective middle ear. In 1974, the National Health Service introduced the behind-the-ear (BE) postaural aids, in which the microphone, amplifier, and receiver are all contained in a small unit that rests on and behind the ear. This type of aid had already been available for a number of years in the private hearing aid sector. An even smaller aid which has recently appeared is the "in-the-ear" aid, in which the whole unit is contained within the ear. This type of aid is not available under the National Health Service. Neither is the spectacle aid, in which the unit is contained in the spectacle arm.[1] Hearing aid refinements include high-tone and low-tone cutouts catering to hearing losses which slope steeply across the frequencies. An automatic volume attenuator can be fitted to a hearing aid for recruitment sufferers.

Sound amplified by a hearing aid will obviously lack the quality of "live" sound. Moreover, for those with sensorineural or "mixed" hearing losses, artificiality caused by amplification will interact with the imperfection of the sensory receptor mechanisms. Almost all hearing aid users also experience considerable difficulty in group situations, or when there is background noise (e.g., in the street or in a busy office). The extent to which hearing aid users are able to learn to habituate to those sounds they do not want to hear, and to selectively attend to those they do want to hear, is not known.

Although the range of aids normally available under the National Health Service has been expanded considerably within the last decade (hearing aid

[1]Certain ear-level NHS aids have adaptors so that they can be fitted to spectacle frames.

companies also offer a wide range of aids), very little is known concerning the matching of hearing aids to hearing impairment. As Moore (1982) puts it:

> there is a paucity of systematic research on which type of aid is best for which type of hearing disorder, and the "prescription" of a hearing aid is often made by inspired guesswork rather than on the basis of sound scientific evidence [p. 254].

Attempts have been made to assess satisfaction with hearing aids. One approach has been to ascertain how much an aid is worn on an "always, often, rarely, never" scale. In general, it has been found that a considerable number of hearing aid owners make little or no use of their aids (Stephens, 1977). However, satisfaction with an aid is not necessarily related to the amount that it is worn. Kapteyn (1977) examined the relationship between items measuring satisfaction with hearing aids and degree of hearing loss. The relationship found was very weak for almost all the items. Kapteyn concluded that the "population consists of subpopulations in which different criteria apply to hearing aid satisfaction . . . these criteria may be more related to psychosocial factors than to technical aspects."

## 2. *Environmental Aids*

A number of appliances, usually known as "environmental aids," are available, full details of which can be obtained from the Royal National Institute for the Deaf, London. The consumer magazine *Which* (October, 1981) has tested many of the aids on the market. A useful television aid, for example, consists of an adaptor which connects the listener directly to the sound source by means of a long lead and an earphone. This enables the listener to receive sound signals free from background noise and allows volume to be adjusted independently of normal television sound output.

Various telephone aids are also available. For those who cannot hear the telephone ring it is possible to obtain bells with increased amplification, an altered frequency, or both. Flashing light systems are also obtainable. In order to aid conversation, amplifiers can be incorporated into the earpiece. An extra earpiece, called a "watch receiver," is also useful; held next to the microphone of a body-worn aid while the handset is held next to the mouth, it can be used to hear incoming speech binaurally. For those who cannot hear anything on the telephone, it can be used by a third person with normal hearing who then repeats the message so that it is understood by the hearing-impaired person, allowing him or her to conduct a telephone conversation.

Other devices include doorbell aids, visual "baby alarms" in which a microphone is connected to a warning light, and alarm clock aids which flash lights or are connected to a vibrator under the pillow. A number of public halls, theatres, and so on are fitted with an induction loop. Hearing aid users can "tune in" to the induction loop and hear speech or music free from background interference.

Despite the wide range of aids available, level of ownership is very low, evidenced by one of the studies to be described later in the book, in which out of a sample of 211 hearing aid owners, 25 had a telephone aid, three a television aid, three a doorbell aid, and two an alarm clock aid.

Recently, attempts have been made to develop systems concentrating on the visual representation of speech, intended mainly for those who obtain little or no benefit from a hearing aid. A telephone package is available in which messages typed by the "speaker" are viewed on a television screen by the "hearer." The video phone also has possibilities for those who are able to supplement limited hearing ability with lipreading. The most far-reaching development, however, concerns verbatim visual transmission of naturally spoken speech. It is very expensive, however, because it involves a third person, a stenographer, who types out an abbreviated form of spoken language which is "read" on a video monitor. This system has been used successfully by a profoundly deaf Member of Parliament. The next step is to develop simultaneous transmission of speech (by using a computer speech reader) and thus do away with the need for a human intermediary.

## H. Statutory and Voluntary Services

The family doctor is normally the first point of contact for someone with a hearing loss. If the doctor thinks it necessary, the person is referred to an ear, nose, and throat surgeon for a thorough investigation, both medical and audiometric. If the hearing loss cannot be treated satisfactorily, a hearing aid is normally recommended. An audiological technician will take an impression for an ear mould and decide on the type of aid most suitable.

At a later appointment the aid is fitted, and the wearer instructed on its use, care, and maintenance. Repairs to aids are carried out at the hospital, which also issues hearing aid batteries free of charge. This brief description covers what is available at present to the vast majority of hearing-impaired people. Following initial contact with a general practitioner, it is of course up to the hearing-impaired person to turn to commercial medicine and to obtain a hearing aid privately if desired.

Some hospitals offer follow-up appointments. A very small number of hospitals have audiological scientists who may participate in hearing aid choice and evaluation. These scientists are usually physicists or engineers with postgraduate training in audiology. Recently, the new post of "hearing therapist" has been created, though few are currently employed in the health service. The role of the hearing therapist is not clearly defined but concentrates on counselling, auditory training, and the teaching of lipreading. A new medical specialisation has also emerged, that of "audiological medicine." These new specialisms reflect a change in the pattern of rehabilitation, partly modelled on provision in Scandinavia, particularly Denmark.

Outside the hospital service, the only professional directly concerned with the welfare of a person with acquired hearing loss is the social worker with the deaf, employed by the Social Services Department of a local authority or by a voluntary organisation. The specialist social worker's main responsibility, however, is with prelingually deaf adults who rely on sign language as a means of communication. Involvement with adults with acquired hearing loss is usually limited to those extremely rare and traumatic instances of severe or profound hearing loss of sudden onset.

While lipreading instruction is widely available, the great majority of classes are provided under the aegis of the Department of Education and Science as evening classes in colleges of further education and evening institutes; the formation and continuance of a class depends on a minimum enrolment and on a teacher who is willing to take on such a class in a part-time capacity. Teachers of lipreading do not have to be qualified teachers or have any other qualification. A 6-week course (at the City Literary Institute Centre for the Deaf, London) is, however, recommended for those who wish to teach lipreading. Other recognised forms of rehabilitation, auditory training, voice conservation, and specialist counselling are virtually unavailable at the present time. For many forms of handicap, residential rehabilitation is available for those who may need it. The only residential facility for adults with acquired hearing loss is run by the Link centre, a voluntary organisation based at Eastbourne. It offers 1- and 2-week courses which can do little more than provide an orientation to rehabilitation.

A number of voluntary organisations exist to promote the interests of those who lose their hearing. The major national organisation is the Royal National Institute for the Deaf. Besides campaigning, the RNID has a well-developed technical department which reports regularly on hearing aids and provides a free (though little publicised) service for the testing of aids. The British Deaf Association is almost exclusively concerned with the prelingually deaf. The British Association of the Hard-of-Hearing is the organisation most directly relevant to those with an acquired hearing loss. Even though it is a national organisation, however, it is poorly endowed, having only one full-time official. The role of the Association is to provide fellowship amongst its members and to coordinate the activities of local societies and clubs.

# CHAPTER TWO

# *Previous Studies*

## I. THE EXPERIENCE OF HEARING LOSS*

### A. Personal Experiences

While acquired hearing loss is relatively common, there are few auto-biographical accounts of its effects. Those that do exist emphasise every-day practical problems associated with hearing loss. Rawson (1973), for example, in an article entitled "The Everyday Consequences of Acquired Deafness," deals with problems caused by background noise, difficulty in location of sound, and the inadequacies of lipreading. She also discusses difficulties associated with travel, and a problem often not appreciated, that of an inability to talk and do something else at the same time, such as eat, walk, or drive, all of which entail taking your eyes away from the speaker's face, thereby losing important visual clues. Jack Ashley, the completely deaf Member of Parliament, has written a book called *Journey into Silence* (Ashley, 1973). The bulk of the book concerns his life before he completely lost his hearing and takes as its theme his political career. Relatively little of the book is devoted to the effects of hearing loss on personal or working relationships. Lysons (1978), in reference to his own hearing loss, shows how he compensated by pursuing academic qualifica-

*Much of this chapter was first published in the form of a review article (Thomas, 1981a).

tions. Savill (1975) graphically describes shortcomings on the part of advisory and professional people in voluntary and governmental organisations with whom she came into contact after completely losing her hearing. It is understandable that autobiographical accounts do not deal at length with the adverse effects of hearing loss on personal well-being. After all, long descriptive accounts of depression or suspicion are difficult to write and are unlikely to have popular appeal. One of the few and perhaps the most well-known accounts of the psychological effects of hearing loss was written by Beethoven (1802). The following extract serves as a succinct rationale for this book. It may be indicative of a general reluctance to admit to psychological stress that Beethoven refused to have the document published during his lifetime. Incidentally, it was written 16 years before the composer became completely deaf (Heiligenstadt Document, from *Letters of Beethoven* by E. Anderson).

> For the last six years, I have been afflicted with the incurable complaint which has been made worse by incompetent doctors. . . . Though endowed with a passionate and lively temperament, and even fond of the distractions offered by society, I was soon obliged to seclude myself and live in solitude. If at times I decided just to ignore my infirmity, alas, how cruelly was I then driven back by the intensified sad experience of my poor hearing. . . . Moreover, my misfortune pains me double, for inasmuch at it leads to my being misjudged. For there can be no relaxation in human society, no refined conversations, no mutual confidences. I must live quite alone and may creep into society only as often as sheer necessity demands. I must live like an outcast. If I appear in company, I am overcome by a burning anxiety, a fear that I am running the risk of letting people notice my condition. . . . Such experiences have almost made me despair, and I was on the point of putting an end to my life— the only thing that held me back was my art.

## B. Clinical Observations

Clinical observers for some considerable time have remarked on the relationship between acquired deafness and psychological disorder. Kraepelin (1915) recorded delusions of persecution amongst people with hearing loss. Haines (1927) maintained that suspicion and depression resulting from isolation were "marked characteristics" resulting from "partial deafness." Today, the two main areas of concern are still the relationship between hearing loss and the neuroses (especially depression) on the one hand, and hearing loss and paranoid mental states on the other. Another early article that seems by its title to be highly relevant is "The Mental Effects of Deafness" (Menninger, 1924). A sentence from this article (often quoted by later writers) states of progressive deafness that: "It is as if something vital to one's existence has been torn from him." The following sentence, however, shows that Menninger wanted to fit deafness into a psychoanalytical framework and was only marginally interested in the phenomenon of hearing loss itself.

> Psychoanalytic study has shown that this deprivation complex (i.e., deafness) has many roots in the unconscious, going back, to give only one example, to the period in early infancy when the nipple was torn from the baby's mouth, a period when the baby made no distinction between its own body and the body of the nipple and bottle or breast [p. 146].

For Menninger, the result of this deprivation was a "sense of inferiority." How this sense of inferiority manifests itself, however, was not explained.

Hunt is one of many otologists to comment on what were presumed to be the drastic effects of hearing loss (Hunt, 1944).

> Fear of failure, fear of ridicule, fear of people, fear of new situations, chance encounters, sudden noises, imagined sounds; fear of being slighted, avoided, made conspicuous; these are but a handful of fears that haunt the waking and even the sleeping hours of the sufferer from progressive deafness. Small wonder that, at best, he tends to live in an atmosphere of despondency and suspicion. Small wonder that, at worst, he may not particularly want to live at all [pp. 230–231].

An important upsurge of interest in the psychological consequences of hearing loss occurred in the years immediately following the Second World War, when the plight of many war-deafened veterans attracted the attention of psychiatrists in the United States. Knapp gives an example of how this came about (Knapp, 1948)

> . . . An abundance of technicians—lip-reading, speech, and acoustic—seemed to make psychiatric assistance superfluous . . . the few cases that did come for consultation were looked on by the psychiatrist as curiosities. Their aberrations were uncritically ascribed to "deafness," as a vague but unitarian entity. The latter assumption gradually dissolved . . . a final fact was that after the first 18 months it became apparent that there were many hysterics in the [deaf] population. More attention began to be devoted to them. During the next half year, the volume of consultations almost tripled. After that, the Psychiatric Service merged informally with the Hearing Service, opened an office on the hearing wards, and worked in complete collaboration with both medical and lay acoustic personnel [pp. 203–204].

Knapp's study of hearing-impaired veterans is fairly typical of many postwar psychiatric reports in that the insights gained are based on the

accumulation of professional experience. Nevertheless, the observations
are revealing and have served to generate useful hypotheses. The majority
of cases seen by Knapp had mild losses, with a minority in the 50- to 80-dB
loss range, and only a tiny fraction with a greater loss. He noted a tendency
for "severe psychiatric reactions to be associated with severe hearing
losses." There was, however, no one "psychology of deafness," but "the
psychology of many individuals defending themselves against a sensory
handicap which led primarily to difficulty in communication." Knapp also
found a tendency for the cases seen to be suspicious, though he was unsure
of the extent to which such suspicion might lead on to paranoid psychosis.
In fact, of all the patients seen, only one case of paranoid psychosis was
diagnosed, and that in a patient with a slight conductive loss. It is important to bear in mind that reactions of hearing-impaired war veterans are
rather untypical, because loss of hearing was almost certainly traumatic.
Moreover, the psychological effect of combat experience might have made
a significant contribution to an abnormal mental state (Knapp, 1948).

Unlike most studies reported soon after the war, a study by Ingalls
(1946) was based on a sample in which the majority had not had combat
experience. "The great majority had partial hearing in one or both ears,"
he wrote. "Most cases were of the chronic, progressive type, with hearing
loss present since childhood." Although not stated explicitly, it seems that
the patients were predominantly young male conscripts. The criterion for
diagnosis of psychoneurosis was "the presence of definite and persistent
symptoms or work inefficiency directly related to early life emotional
conflicts." Ingalls reported that "the great majority of the neuroses were
of the anxiety type. Hysteria, depression, and psychosomatic symptoms
were frequent complicating features. Four instances of psychosis were
observed, one of these patients had a severe depression from which he
recovered following the fitting of a hearing aid. Another suffered from
dementia praecox, paranoid type (Ingalls, 1946)."

Ramsdell (1962) also treated World War II veterans. He found depression and suspicion to be the most common symptoms. Ramsdell went
further than the description of cases, however, and examined what he
believed to be the special relationship between hearing and psychological
well-being. He postulated three levels of hearing: symbolic, warning, and
background. Ramsdell argued that the importance of the background level
had not generally been recognised, "although it is psychologically the

most fundamental of auditory functions." The background sounds which constituted what he described as the primitive level of hearing changed constantly "because the world around us in a constant state of activity . . . [hence] the primitive function of hearing maintains a readiness to react by keeping us constantly informed of events about us. It also contributes to our sense of comfort by ever reassuring us that we are part of the living, ongoing world." Based on observations of very many patients, Ramsdell was convinced that common depressive reactions resulted from an interference with the primitive level of hearing. He quoted a typical patient who asked, "Why am I so depressed, so caught in a dead world?" Ramsdell did not believe that loss of function at the warning or symbolic levels was as important as loss at the primitive level, for it would not be so all-pervading. These speculations, while interesting, have no basis over and above their intuitive appeal. Nevertheless, Ramsdell's three levels of hearing have been quoted by numerous writers as if they had a solid theoretical validity.

Levine, in a book concerned mainly with prelingual deafness, devoted a chapter to the hard-of-hearing, consisting mainly of practical advice for those who come into contact with the hearing impaired. The following quotation from a teacher of lipreading illustrates the dramatic effect which hearing loss may have on a person's life (Levine, 1960):

> Threats of suicide, rage, depression, isolation, self-hate, shame, and suspicion are part of her daily contacts with her pupils as they go through the period of intense emotional struggle due to sudden loss of hearing or sudden realisation that the handicap is permanent or progressive [p. 62].

Levine summarised the problems of living with hearing loss as follows:

> Where the individual is accustomed to be an integral part of a close relationship, as in the family, on the job, and in the community, to be suddenly left alone is tantamount to ostracism. It is not surprising, therefore, to find many such persons engulfed in torments of despair, panic, rage, and a feeling of worthlessness . . . the naive and well-intentioned efforts of family and friends to cheer up such a person may add just enough extra irritation to an already overburdened psyche to cause emotional collapse [p. 65].

John Denmark has argued that children have an "amazing resilience and often readily adjust to the onset of deafness, while onset in adult life affects the whole lifestyle of the individual . . . and results in severe psychiatric illness." In support of this, he quotes two typical case studies, one of progressive and one of sudden hearing loss, in which both subjects complained of intense depression. Denmark also believed that "suspicion and hostility are not uncommon, especially in sensitive personalities, but the commonest feelings are those of isolation, insecurity, and depression" (Denmark, 1976).


## C.  Simulation Studies

To date, there have been no systematic studies of the effects of an experimentally induced hearing loss, mainly because of the technical difficulties involved. Simulation in a laboratory setting poses few problems but is obviously far removed from real-life situations. The simplest device is the ear plug, but the resulting decrement of 30 dB at most is little more than marginal, at least for those who have normal hearing to start with. Even so, the effects produced may be considerable. Hebb *et al.* (1954) paid six college students to spend a weekend with their ears packed with cotton impregnated with petroleum jelly. They were given no information about expected results, but were expected to keep a diary. Two of the subjects reported only trivial emotional effects. One reported strong feelings of personal inadequacy but denied irritability—his girlfriend disagreed and described him as irritable and withdrawn during the whole experiment. The other three reported emotional reactions, especially of irritability and withdrawal. One of them, a male, complained of sleep disturbance and inability to concentrate. Another, the only female in the group, commented that "I feel that this lack of hearing is giving me a snivelling personality." Co-workers believed that these three appeared "to present evidence of a slight personality disturbance."

It seems that the introduction of a masking noise into the ears is the only method by which a marked hearing loss can be simulated. Even this method is limited, however, because if the masking noise is too loud, it is likely to be heard by other people. Lieth (1972a) reports an experiment in which he spent a few days wearing a noise generator connected to a binaural hearing aid which resulted in a hearing decrement roughly equivalent to 50 dB. The generator which Lieth had strapped to his back was rather cumbersome and may possibly have contributed, along with noise, to the heightened irritability he reported. The main effect described by

Lieth was what he termed *social deafness,* which referred to the difficulties he encountered in group conversations. Lieth also reported that his family became increasingly irritable. He also found that he was unable to refrain from invading other people's personal space. Perhaps the most objective evidence for the stress caused by hearing loss was that he was forced to turn the device off on two occasions of family crisis!

Simulation studies can be expected to improve. Stephens (1982), for example, reports simulation of moderate to severe hearing loss with the combined use of earplugs and tinnitus maskers.

## II. EXPERIMENTAL STUDIES

### A. Welles (1932)

A number of studies reported in the 1930s have been reviewed by Barker *et al.* (1953). The most systematic of these, based on the Bernreuter Personality Inventory, was carried out by Welles (1932). The respondents in Welles's study were members of organisations for the hard-of-hearing. A matched control group was formed by asking the hard-of-hearing to give a copy of the Inventory to a hearing friend of the same sex and approximately the same age, education, and social status. In all, 528 pairs of questionnaires were distributed. A total of 225 (43%) questionnaires were returned by the hard-of-hearing group, and 148 (28%) by the control group. Eighty-seven percent of the hard-of-hearing and 89% of the control group responders were women.

The results of the study were analysed in two ways. Firstly, the scores of the experimental and control groups were compared. The hard-of-hearing, experimental group was found to be significantly more emotional, more introverted, and less dominant than the average of their hearing friends. On a measure of self-sufficiency, however, there was no difference. Secondly, a group representing 16% of the hard-of-hearing responders was selected on the basis of "having successfully surmounted their handicap." When this subsample was compared with the matched control group, no differences were found on any of the Bernreuter scales. While mean differences for the control and experimental groups taken as a whole were significant, the degree of overlap on all measures led Welles to conclude that the hard-of-hearing are only slightly more emotional, introverted, and submissive than normal. Those who had achieved success in life, despite hearing loss, did not differ from the control group in their scores on the Bernreuter Personality Inventory.

The diagnostic significance of certain items in psychological inventories constitutes a problem which has beset the study of hearing impairment. In their review of early studies, based on the Bernreuter Personality Inventory, Barker and his associates argued that the inventory contained many items "predisposed in one direction by a hearing impairment, regardless of their intended psychological significance." Welles was not unaware of the problem of the validity of the Inventory for people with a hearing loss. In order to find out if such items had led to misclassification, he selected the 16 items which best discriminated between the experimental and control groups. They describe the hard-of-hearing group as follows (Welles, 1932):

1. More often easily discouraged when the opinions of others differ from their own.
2. Less often find conversation more helpful in formulating their ideas than reading.
3. Less often prefer a play to a dance.
4. Less often careful in not saying things to hurt other people's feelings.
5. Less often heckle or question a public speaker.
6. More often feel reluctant at a reception or tea to meet the most important person present.
7. Less often see more fun or humour in things when they are in a group than when alone.
8. More often find books more entertaining than companions.
9. More often have ever had spells of dizziness.
10. More often feel lonesome when they are with other people.
11. More often have frequently appeared as a lecturer or entertainer before groups of people.
12. Less often find people more stimulating to them than anything else.
13. More often have difficulty in starting a conversation with a stranger.
14. More often get as many ideas at the time of reading a book as they do from a discussion of it afterward.
15. Less often face their troubles alone without seeking help.
16. More often optimistic when others about them are greatly depressed [p. 66].

Welles then asked a number of psychologists and executives of a league for the hard-of-hearing to point to any items in the Inventory which they felt were biased for the hard-of-hearing. He found, intriguingly, that "a majority of each group of judges marked only 3 of these 16 significant items, there being no complete agreement on any one item in either group.'' Welles then argued that the finding were in no way invalidated by these three items because when they were removed, the significant differences between the experimental and control groups remained unaltered. However, as Barker and his associates commented (Barker *et al.*, 1953)

> . . . a number of other items might easily reflect the sensory handicap apart from its psychological significance for behaviour, although, as has been noted, only three such items were agreed upon by a majority of judges [p. 217].

It seems, therefore, that the problem of misclassification was not adequately controlled. The validity of the findings is also in question because the sample is unlikely to be representative, not so much because of the low response rate and massive sex bias, but because few hearing-impaired people join societies for the hard-of-hearing. In one of the studies to be described later in the book, only 2 out of a total sample of 211 people contacted through NHS Hearing Aid Clinics were members of organisations for the hard-of-hearing. This was the first study of hearing loss based on a large and relatively unbiased sample.

## B. Nett (1960)

Nett's study is little known and rarely quoted, probably because it exists as an unpublished report. The study was ''directed toward determining among adult individuals the social–psychological–vocational handicapping which results from hearing loss.'' Nett interviewed 378 respondents who were attending an audiology clinic, having been referred from private practitioners and a hospital outpatient department, or who, in some cases, were self-referred. Those who volunteered to take part in the project were interviewed immediately after audiological examination. Nearly half (43%) appear to have had normal or very near normal hearing (mean loss of 29 dB or less).

Nett administered two psychological inventories, the WAIS (Wechsler Adult Intelligence Scale) and the MMPI (Minnesota Multiphasic Personality Inventory). For what it is worth, the mean IQ of the sample was 104. With regard to the MMPI, Nett concluded that scores on certain scales differed significantly from standardised norms. The MMPI appears only to have been administered to 133 patients, 51 (38%) of whom had normal hearing with a loss of 29 dB or less. About 20% of the patients scored outside the normal range (18% for the Depression Scale). (The scale which showed the least deviation from normal was the Paranoia Scale!) It seems, therefore, that this section of the sample was emotionally disturbed. However, almost all of the participants were patients at the time of administration of the MMPI. Uncertainty about diagnosis and anxiety associated with hospital attendance might have contributed to the elevated scores. Moreover, as patients were being referred for consideration for hearing-aid fitting, it is fair to assume that hearing loss was in almost all cases untreated. Given the universal availability of hearing aids, at least in the United Kingdom, it would seem that the most appropriate time to measure the effect of hearing loss is some time after the fitting of an aid.

A remarkable aspect of Nett's study concerns her claim that MMPI scores can be predicted from mean dB loss. The correlations are based on 133 patients (Table 2.1). Nett stated that the correlation coefficient *ETA* was selected "because we were not sure that linear relationships would be the rule, and the correlation ratio is a good index when a curved regression prevails." Nett provided one scattergram, for the relationship between depression and weighted dB loss (Table 2.2A). The ETA coefficient obtained was 0.78. While such a coefficient is statistically highly significant, there does not seem to be, on visual inspection, a curvilinear or any other form of relationship between the two variables. It seems as if Nett has

TABLE 2.1

How Well Can We Predict MMPI Scores from Hearing Loss?[a]

| Hearing loss measures | ETA coefficients[b] | | | | |
|---|---|---|---|---|---|
|  | hs | d | hy | pa | si |
| Speech reception threshold | 52[c] | 51[c] | 56[c] | 56[c] | 57[c] |
| Speech discrimination | 36 | 42[c] | 33 | 49[c] | 39 |
| Weighted % dB loss | 71[c] | 78[c] | 72[c] | 79[c] | 77[c] |
| Social Adequacy Index | 73[c] | 74[c] | 78[c] | 74[c] | 71[c] |

[a]From Nett, 1960; $N = 133$.

[b]Decimal points excluded. Abbreviations: hs, hypochondriasis; d, depression; hy, hysteria; pa, paranoia; si, social introversion.

[c]$p < .05$.

TABLE 2.2A

Scattergram for Relationship between Weighted dB Loss and the Depression Scale of the MMPI[a]

| Weighted dB loss | Depression score | | | | | |
|---|---|---|---|---|---|---|
| | 30–39 | 40–49 | 50–59 | 60–69 | 70–79 | 80–89 |
| 90–100 | | 1 | 1 | 2 | | |
| 80–89 | | 1 | | 1 | 1 | |
| 70–79 | | | | 4 | | 2 |
| 60–69 | | 4 | 2 | 2 | 1 | |
| 50–59 | 4 | 3 | 6 | 5 | 2 | 2 |
| 40–49 | 1 | 5 | 4 | 3 | 1 | |
| 30–39 | 3 | 1 | 7 | 9 | 2 | 2 |
| 20–29 | | 6 | 6 | 9 | 6 | 1 |
| 10–19 | 1 | 3 | 8 | 3 | | 1 |
| 1–9 | | 2 | 3 | 1 | | 1 |

[a]From Nett, 1960; $N = 133$.

chosen ETA for the wrong reason and obtained a spuriously high degree of relationship. There is certainly not an *a priori* reason for expecting any systematic form of variation which is nonlinear. Neither does the scattergram reveal any such relationship. Moreover, Nett does not offer any interpretation concerning the nature of the relationship. On the assumption that weighted dB loss and a standardised measure of depression are both normally distributed, a Pearson Product Moment Correlation was calculated based on an analysis of the grouped data in Table 2.2A. The resulting correlation coefficient was 0.01. This, of course, could disguise a curvilinear relationship if one existed. There was no discernible relationship in the scattergram, however; neither does one emerge if the mean depression score is calculated for different degrees of hearing loss (Table 2.2B). It is obvious from the re-analysis that the use of an ETA coefficient as opposed to a parametric coefficient was mistaken. An ETA coefficient is calculated from grouped data. It is designed to detect a nonlinear relationship, if one exists. It does this by maximising any form of relationship which the data describe. Hence, if raw data are used, the relationship will be one of unity because the exact relationship between the two variables will have been described. It follows from this that an analysis based on a large number of groups will also yield an inflated coefficient, as was the case with Nett.

TABLE 2.2B

Mean Depression Scores Calculated from the Scattergram

| | Weighted dB loss | | | | | | | | | |
|---|---|---|---|---|---|---|---|---|---|---|
| | 1–9 | 10–19 | 20–29 | 30–39 | 40–49 | 50–59 | 60–69 | 70–79 | 80–89 | 90–100 |
| Mean depression scores | 60 | 55 | 61 | 60 | 53 | 56 | 55 | 71 | 61 | 57 |
| N | 7 | 16 | 28 | 24 | 14 | 22 | 9 | 6 | 3 | 4 |

[a]From Nett, 1960; N = 133.

Had the number of groups on which the calculations were based been fewer, the ETA would have been reduced markedly (for further details of the misuse of correlation coefficients such as ETA, see Mueller *et al.*, 1970). Nett provided detailed data for the Depression Scale only, and so it was not possible for me to ascertain how the other coefficients given in Tables 2.2A and 2.2B were obtained. It seems fair to assume that they are inflated in the same way as is the coefficient for the realtionship between depression and severity of hearing loss (Table 2.2).

### C.  Myklebust (1964)

Myklebust administered the MMPI to hard-of-hearing adults belonging to a New York Hearing Society concerned with lipreading and various other activities. The sample consisted of 44 males (mean age 40) and 83 females (mean age 50). Mean hearing loss was 66 dB, and the mean age of onset was 18 for men and 24 for women. Despite what might be expected from the age of the respondents, only 34% of the men and 24% of the women were married. Myklebust reported significantly elevated scores on all the MMPI scales with the exception of Paranoia. He then attempted to take into account eight MMPI items which are "loaded" for "the hearing impaired because they refer specifically to hearing, speech, or balance." Here, by way of example, are three of them:

> My hearing is apparently as good as most people's.
> I have no difficulty in keeping my balance when walking
> I do not often notice my ears ringing or buzzing.

Exclusion of the eight items from the analysis did not affect the overall profile. However, other items which could conceivably be loaded by virtue of their social nature (there are many in the MMPI) were not considered. Moreover, the use of a hearing society as a sampling source has already been queried in relation to Welles's study (described above). The sample seems further biased toward the unattached, particularly women. In fact, Myklebust found that "the group of hard-of-hearing females who were married were better adjusted emotionally." However, the study does demonstrate that adults who join a society for the hard-of-hearing may indeed be emotionally disturbed, if only because Depression scale scores which do not contain loaded items were particularly elevated. Thus, while the sample may not be representative of the hard-of-hearing population, its members do appear to constitute a group which sought the support and counselling they almost certainly did not receive when they bought their hearing aids.

### D. Mahapatra (1974a,b)

Mahapatra tested the hypothesis that a group with bilateral hearing loss would suffer greater psychiatric disturbance than a unilaterally impaired control group. His sample consisted of 89 otosclerotic patients consecutively admitted to the ENT ward of a general infirmary for stapedectomy. Not one of the patients had any kind of psychiatric history. They were divided into an experimental group of 49 patients (25 females, 24 males) who were bilaterally impaired with a hearing loss in excess of 40 dB in the better ear, and a unilaterally impaired control group of 40 patients (16 females, 24 males) with a hearing loss in excess of 40 dB in the worse ear. Hearing loss was calculated at 250 Hz only. The mean ages of the groups were 45 and 43, with standard deviations between 11 and 12. On the day prior to the operation, each patient completed the Cornell Index, a psychiatric screening inventory. This was followed immediately by a psychiatric interview with Mahapatra. The mean Cornell Index scores for the two groups were 14.7 (SD 11.5) for the experimental group, and 7.9 (SD 6.1) for the control group. The difference between these means was statistically significant. Overall, females scored significantly higher than males. The Cornell Index consists of 101 items. The cutoff score suggested by its authors for discrimination between normals and non-normals is 13. A comparison of the two groups with reference to this cutoff point is given in Table 2.3. Once again, the difference is highly significant.

As stated above, administration of the Cornell Index was followed by a standard psychiatric interview with the author. At the time of the interview, Mahapatra was unaware of the Cornell Index Scores. Overall, the findings based on the psychatric inventory confirmed those obtained with the Cornell Index with regard to differences between the two groups. Moreover, there was a high degree of agreement between the Cornell Index Score and the clinical interview at the individual level, at least for the 24 "deaf" patients diagnosed as psychiatrically disturbed, 18 of whom had a Cornell Index score of 13 or over. No information is given concerning

TABLE 2.3

Cornell Index Scores of Hearing Impaired and Control Groups[a]

| Cornell Index Scores | Males[b] | | Females[c] | | Total[d] | |
|---|---|---|---|---|---|---|
| | deaf | controls | deaf | controls | deaf | controls |
| <13 | 26 | 21 | 9 | 12 | 35 | 33 |
| ≥13 | 8 | 3 | 16 | 4 | 24 | 7 |

[a]From Mahapatra, 1974a,b.
[b]NS.
[c]$p < .005$.
[d]$p < .005$.

agreement between interview and Cornell Index for the control group. Of the 10 patients with losses in excess of 70 dB, 5 had a Cornell Index score of 13 or more, but only 2 were diagnosed as psychiatrically ill at the subsequent interviews.

The research design for this study is ingenious, and appears to illustrate a strong link between hearing loss and psychiatric disturbance. Unfortunately, there are a number of serious weaknesses. Firstly, there are numerous items in the inventory which might misclassify psychologically normal people who are hearing impaired. While it is possible that Mahapatra was aware of the danger of misclassifying hearing-impaired people, he did not refer to it, nor did he attempt any form of item analysis.

The second and third points concern the apparent lack of knowledge of hearing loss on the part of the author. This is not to say that a researcher need necessarily be an expert in any area he chooses to investigate. In this case, however, the lack of understanding has resulted in poor research design and misleading interpretation. Poor research design results from using the frequency of 250 Hz only. This frequency is outside the speech range and has little significance for understanding of speech. Normal practice is to take 1 kilohertz (kHz) as a single frequency, or the mean or weighted mean of three or more of 0.5, 1, 2, 3, and 4 kHz. Moreover, measurement of hearing at 250 Hz may be unreliable, because it is susceptible to masking by ambient noise unless the testing situation is extremely good (Martin *et al.*, 1971). Misleading interpretation arises in the discussion of results where Mahapatra concludes that his findings ''are contrary to the conclusion Furth (1966) drew when he reported that the adult deaf did not differ in any way from the adult with normal hearing.'' Mahapatra does not grasp that Furth is referring to the prelingually "deaf" and noting that despite their very poor language and educational attainment, they still somehow grow up, get married (and divorced), have children, steady jobs, mortgages, and so on. The point Furth wishes to make is that the growth of thought processes without the aid of normal language (the reference refers to his book, *Thinking without Language*) nevertheless results in a normal ability to cope with the exigencies of adult life, and that this is best explained in terms of Piagetian formulations, in which the growth of intelligence is seen to be largely independent of oral language development.

Finally, Mahapatra's patients were examined on the day prior to surgery, which for those with bilateral hearing loss would be critical in its consequences. The unilaterally impaired control group had functionally normal or near-normal hearing; for these patients, successful surgery would result in minor improvement in hearing only. Hence, the difference between the two groups, while valid, could simply reflect an artefactual relationship to hearing loss, the main causal factor being concern over critical surgery and not the experience of living with hearing loss.

Incidentally, Mahapatra diagnosed five patients as paranoid schizophrenics, a finding discussed later in this chapter.

## E.  Other Studies

Gildston and Gildston (1972) examined personality changes associated with surgically corrected conductive hearing loss. The Guilford-Zimmerman Temperament Survey (Guilford and Zimmerman, 1949) was administered two or three weeks before, and three months after, surgery to a group of 34 hard-of-hearing patients. They found on first administration of the inventory that the patients displayed negative qualities relating to the traits of ascendance, sociability, emotional stability, and objectivity when compared with the normally hearing population. Post-operative measures, however, showed significant changes towards normality on all traits. Moreover, five patients for whom the operation did not restore normal hearing did not display changes towards normality.

Stephens (1980) administered the Eysenck Personality Inventory and the Crown-Crisp Experiential Index (Crown and Crisp, 1979) to 353 hearing-impaired patients who were consecutive attenders at the Audiology Unit of the Institute of Sound and Vibration Research at the University of Southampton. The group as a whole was found to be significantly introverted and neurotic when compared with the normal population. The group also deviated significantly (in the predicted direction) from the norms on all but one of the scales of the Experiental Index (obsessionality, anxiety, phobic anxiety, somatic preoccupation, and depression). The exception was the hysteria scale. The most pronounced deviation was for the anxiety scale. The characteristics of the sample were not described. Nor can it be known to what extent the sample, obtained from a specialised research unit, was representative of adults with acquired hearing loss. Moreover, deviations from norms, while statistically significant, were not very large, with the possible exception of the anxiety scale of the Experiental Index. It is also possible that unusual problem cases, as most of the group were, would be more likely to be psychologically disturbed. With regard to this latter point, Stephens informs me that many patients were referred to the Unit in order to differentiate between Ménière's disorder and VIIIth nerve tumours. Hence, a sizable proportion would have suffered from Ménière's disorder, which is known to have a significant psychosomatic component, and thus could account for the elevated scores obtained (Stephens, 1982).

Weir and Stephens (1976), in a study of ENT outpatients, found that patients with a sensorineural hearing loss ($N = 11$) did not differ significantly from other classes of ENT outpatients with respect to Crown-Crisp Experiental Index scores ($N = 159$).

Cattell et al. (1970) reported the administration of the 16PF to groups of subjects with certain physical disabilities, including a group of 37 people who were "deaf" or had "serious" hearing disorders. Given that the hearing-impaired group was found to be "duller" than any of the other groups, one might speculate that the group was partly composed of pre-lingually deaf subjects who are known to underachieve on tests of verbal ability. Apart from this, the group as a whole turned out to be more shy, sensitive, and submissive than the other groups, yet at the same time more shrewd, astute, and socially aware. Clearly, little confidence can be placed in such contradictory findings based on an ill-defined sample.

### III.  HEARING LOSS AND PARANOID MENTAL STATES

Suspiciousness is traditionally associated with hearing loss. Paranoid mental states may, but do not necessarily, include delusions in which suspiciousness is a major component. The logical leap is obvious. If hearing-impaired individuals are more suspicious than normal, they are also more likely to be paranoid. Consider Phillips and Rowell (1932), for example:

> What a nuisance they [the hearing impaired] are, we think. So we ostracise them cruelly. They can't help becoming introverts . . . from introversion to paranoia is no long step. The shut-in individual may easily develop a twisted philosophy of life based on persecution. The asocial traits appear [p. 148].

Or Levine (1960):

> While deafness does not itself produce mental illness, it does by its very nature provoke paranoid ideas in sensitive individuals by keeping them from direct contact with what others in the environment are saying and thinking, thus laying the foundation for suspicion [p. 246].

Or Markides *et al.* (1979):

> . . . suspicion of friends and family, over-sensitivity, irritability, and sometimes an acute state of paranoia are well-known psychological by-products of hearing impairment in adults. . . . (Official policy statement of the British Society of Audiology)

Contrary to popular belief, evidence in support of the presumed association between hearing loss and paraniod mental states is weak. The studies which have been carried out are of two kinds, based on hearing-impaired and paraniod samples. These will now be considered.

### A.  Samples of the Hearing Impaired

Psychiatrists working with war-deafened veterans reported no more than a handful of paranoid cases amongst thousands of referrals (Ingalls, 1946; Knapp, 1948; Ramsdell, 1962). In fact, Knapp pointed out that when "ideas of reference" were present, "they often appeared practical and realistic rather than delusional."

Cooper (1976) noted that there was little agreement amongst researchers concerning the incidence of paranoid reactions in hearing-impaired samples, acknowledging that Knapp and Ingalls had found such reactions to be extremely rare. On the other hand, Cooper quoted Ramsdell (1962), Denmark (1969), and Mahapatra (1974a) as authors who had "commented on the morbid suspiciousness and hostility in these patients, some of whom were frankly psychotic." However, the only reference which Denmark makes to paranoia is to state that "suspicion and hostility are not uncommon experiences in sensitive personalities." Ramsdell similarly gives little space to paranoid reactions. After making a point similar to Denmark's, he qualified it by saying that the term *paranoia* "is often used, perhaps erroneously, to characterise the hypersensitivity of the deaf." Interestingly, when Myklebust (1964) administered the MMPI to members of a New York society for the hard-of-hearing, the Paranoia Scale was the only one which did not clearly differentiate the hearing-impaired group from the general population. Nett (1960) also reported that the Paranoia Scale of the MMPI was the one which deviated least from norms. This leaves Mahapatra's study as the only one which has reported actual cases of paranoid psychosis in samples of hearing-impaired people.

Mahapatra's study has already been discussed at length in relation to general psychological disturbance. Of the 49 hearing-impaired patients who were administered a standard psychiatric interview, five were diagnosed as "paranoid schizophrenics," none of whom had any previous psychiatric history, most of whom had mild conductive losses, and all of whom were about to undergo surgery which had a very high probability of success. The shortcomings of this study, discussed earlier, had to do with research design and not clinical judgement. It is highly unlikely that an experienced clinician would not take into account the danger of misdiagnosis resulting from mistakenly attributing the behavioural effects of hearing loss to underlying psychological causes. On the other hand, Mahapatra's is the *only* study of hearing-impaired samples in which a number of cases of paranoid psychosis have supposedly been found.

Finally, Zimbardo and Andersen (1981) found that six subjects made partially "deaf" by self-hypnosis, but kept unaware of the source of their deafness, became instantly more paranoid than six subjects who were aware of the source of their deafness.

## B.  Paranoid Samples


A different approach has entailed the measurement of hearing loss in samples of psychiatric patients already diagnosed as suffering from paranoid psychoses. Since Kraepelin (1915) first reported such a case, a number of investigators have noted the presence of hearing loss in such patients (Houston and Royse, 1954; Kay and Roth, 1961; Post, 1966; McClelland *et al.*, 1968). However, in none of these studies was the role of hearing loss investigated systematically. As Cooper *et al.* (1974) pointed out, "hearing loss was only one factor among many examined, its duration was not always determined . . . actual hearing loss was not measured, and no otological diagnoses were made."

Two studies have attempted a more systematic examination of the part played by hearing loss in paranoid reactions. In the first (Cooper *et al.*, 1974; Kay *et al.*, 1976), "social deafness" was found "to be one of a number of premorbid characteristics which independently discriminates between groups of patients with paranoid and affective psychoses." Other characteristics were a "schizoid personality" factor, the number of surviving children, precipitating events, family history, and social class. All the factors, taken together, predicted 40% of the variance, implying that the part played by hearing loss may be rather small. Moreover, the mean hearing loss for the paranoid group was 41 dB, and for the affective group, 31 dB, both very mild, and only minimally different from each other. In fact, both could be defined as marginal losses. Even this small difference in hearing sensitivity between the two groups can equally be explained in terms of social class membership, 56% of the paranoid and 30% of the affective group belonging to social classes IV and V. The greater mean hearing loss in the paranoid group, therefore, might simply be explained in terms of poorer general health and/or exposure to industrial noise, both of which are known to be more prevalent in lower socioeconomic groups (Davis, 1983). Another possibility which could easily account for such a small difference in hearing loss is that reliability of audiometric measurement may be differentially affected according to psychiatric diagnosis. Stephens (1973), for example, has shown how certain personality factors influence hearing measurement. Yet again, hearing loss encountered in samples which are psychologically abnormal could be non-organic (Chaiklin & Ventry, 1963). While non-organic hearing loss may be disabling, it will almost certainly be the result of psychosis, rather than the cause of it.

The second study was based on a psychiatric population in New Delhi (Mahendru *et al.*, 1978). Mahendru and his associates compared 67 patients found to have a bilateral hearing loss of >40 dB (once again at 250 Hz only) with 1549 patients whose hearing was normal according to this criterion. The main demographic difference between the two groups was, as expected, a massive age difference, the hearing impaired group being markedly older. With regard to psychiatric diagnosis, 302 (19.5%) of the normally hearing and 37 (55.3%) of the hearing impaired were classified as schizophrenic. Within this subtype, 47 (15.5%) and 21 (64.8%) in the normally hearing and hearing-impaired groups, respectively, were further classified as paranoid. Thus, those with a hearing impairment were four times as likely to be classified as paranoid. Unfortunately, the extent to which the differences between the subsamples could be explained by factors other than hearing loss (e.g., social class, age) was not explored. Nor was the actual difference in degree of hearing loss between the two subsamples calculated.

To conclude, the generally accepted belief in an association between hearing loss and paranoid mental states is unsubstantiated on the basis of evidence currently available.

What is often not appreciated is the effect that hearing loss may have on the diagnosis and treatment of psychiatric patients in general. Denmark, for example, has suggested that "psychiatrists often fail to appreciate in a particular case the benefits which may accrue from otological examination and treatment" (Denmark, 1969). Jeter (1976) reported a study in which 221 psychiatric patients were screened for hearing loss. In all, 18% could not be tested. Of the rest, 60 were screened as hearing impaired, underlining the need for routine audiological examination of psychiatric patients in general.

## IV.  SOCIAL ASPECTS

Given the obvious adverse effects which hearing loss has on conversation, it is surprising how little attention has been devoted to family and social life, and to the effect of hearing impairment at work.

As part of her study of the relationship between audiological measures and handicap, Nett (1960) examined the effect of hearing loss on employment and social and family life, both from the patients' point of view and from that of family, friends, and employers. The data obtained were for the most part restricted to "critical incidents," or specific and observable behavioural acts related to "auditory failure." These were obtained from answers to the open-ended question: Can you tell us how your hearing loss affects your everyday life? Auditory failure was defined as "failing to hear, understand, or localise an auditory stimulus. In a large proportion of "critical instances," the hearing-impaired person was not aware of his failure to receive an auditory stimulus, for example, answer the telephone or doorbell, or reply to a question. In other cases, someone interceded on his or her behalf. Typical responses to "auditory failure" when the hearing-impaired person knew that he had failed to hear are given in Table 2.4.

Nett's 1960 study includes first-hand testimony describing some of the instances in detail.

> "Everyday, I take a fella back and forth to work in my car. I can't hear him well at all; he has a low voice. . . . I turn up the car radio, then he has to talk louder, and then I can hear [p. 65]."

> "The last time I went to a dance, which was about two weeks ago, I was dancing with somebody else's wife. I was carrying on, or trying to carry on, a little conversation. I get embarrassed because I can't hear what she is saying. There's too much noise from the orchestra and people around you. You just don't hear a person that's talking softly next to you. . . . You do what a lot of people who are hard-of-hearing do without realising it—you talk, rather than listen . . . you become a bore [p. 65]."

> "I was at my brother's house last night. There was some conversation I didn't hear. I had to guess when to laugh. A couple of times I guessed wrong [p. 65]."

> "Today at work all the fellows were eating lunch together. I just can't hear well in a bunch like that. I went over by myself and ate . . . this happens almost everyday [p. 68]."

Nett also classified consequences of the critical incidents. They fell roughly into four groups, which in rank order of importance were

1. Suffers self-damage (embarrassed, made to appear foolish or stupid)
   Feels anger towards self
   Avoids situations
   Feels angry with someone else
2. Feels hostility of others
   Argues or upsets someone else

## TABLE 2.4

Typical Responses to Auditory Failure (When the
Hearing-Impaired Person Knows He or She Has Failed
to Hear)[a]

| Response | % |
| --- | --- |
| Ask for repetition | 28 |
| Obtain assistance | 14 |
| Pretend, guess, or bluff | 14 |
| Intentionally do nothing | 12 |
| Get into a better position | 9 |
| Make a mechanical adaptation | 8 |
| Ask for repetition and get into a better position | 4 |
| Withdraw | 4 |
| Tell about loss beforehand | 3 |
| Depend on sight | 2 |
| Read lips | 2 |

[a]From Nett, 1960.

Feels unconcerned
Job affected in some way
3. Withdraws from conversation
Withdraws physically
Makes arrangements for future situations
Suffers mental strain
4. Inconveniences someone
Feels others unaware of what it is like to be hard-of-hearing
Participation limited or prevented (e.g., stopped attending meetings, refused to accept an office, did not go to a party)
Life endangered.

Myklebust obtained autobiographical accounts of the social effects of hearing loss. Most participants described their families as helpful and sympathetic, although they recognised that a great deal of patience on the part of normally hearing members was required. Dependency was emphasised, especially with regard to messages, seeking employment, and maintaining friendships. A finding which struck Myklebust as surprising was that very few had kept the same friends they had had prior to the onset of hearing loss (Myklebust, 1964).

The social isolation resulting from impaired hearing was markedly apparent. Some found the loss of their old friends one of the greatest hardships associated with deafness, and because of this experience many were despondent [p. 131].

This finding may be restricted, of course, to the very small number of people who join clubs for the hard-of-hearing (see page 35), and whose reason for joining may well have been the loss of friends.

The only study of employment problems known to me is an unpublished report (submitted to the United Kingdom Department of Health and Social Security) of a project examining communication patterns among hearing-impaired clerical workers (Bird and Trevains, 1978). The main conclusion was that the 33 clerical workers who took part engaged in less face-to-face communication and relied more on the written word. In general, they had lower expectations for advancement, a finding which the authors believed to be the explanation for the rather surprising finding concerning a high level of job satisfaction. Colleagues and employers in general were sympathetic and helpful.

No research has been undertaken on the effect of hearing loss on family life.

# PART TWO

*The First Study*

# CHAPTER THREE

*Methodology and Audiological Characteristics*

## I. METHODOLOGY

### A. The Sample

The main purpose of this study was to examine the effects of hearing loss on adults of employment age who had owned a hearing aid for a minimum of 1 year. A sample was drawn from NHS hearing aid clinics in the Greater London area, north of the Thames. The original intention of drawing a representative sample from all the clinics in the catchment area had to be abandoned for a number of reasons, among them unsuitable methods of record keeping, lacking of interviewing facilities, and sometimes even a lack of cooperation. The outcome was that the final sample of 211 was drawn from three clinics which would at least provide a characteristic London sample, one at a Central London teaching hospital, and two at general hospitals in the inner and outer suburbs.

The target sample consisted of adults of employment age (16 to 64 for men and 16 to 59 for women) who had been issued a hearing aid for the first time since 1970, and who had owned a hearing aid for a minimum of 1 year. All types and degrees of hearing loss were included. While opinion differed as to whether those with conductive losses should be included, there is no evidence that conductive hearing loss does not have adverse social and psychological consequences. The same reasoning held for the inclusion of those with marginal losses. In fact, a number of writers have argued that a slight hearing loss can be just as disturbing as a severe one (e.g., Myklebust, 1964; Lieth, 1972b).

Although the aim was to interview all those in the three hearing aid clinics who fulfilled the criteria for inclusion in the sample, a number of factors prevented this. Unbeknown to us at the time, one clinic had excluded those cases, admittedly very few, who had not been given a hearing aid because they were deemed to be too deaf to make any use of it. In another, the senior ENT consultant himself carried out the selection of prospective respondents with the specific intention of excluding those with serious social and psychological problems, because he believed they should not be interviewed by nonmedical personnel. In both cases, any resulting bias should be contra-hypothesis, that is, in the direction of less, rather than greater, stress.

The final sample of 211 represented a response rate of 48%, which is reasonably good for this type of study (cf. Bird & Trevains, 1978; McCormick, 1980; Watts *et al.*, 1980). Haggard *et al.* (1981b) report that response rates of between 30 and 40% are typical when patients are asked to revisit a clinic for further testing.

The likely response rate became known at the time of the pilot study, when out of the 40 people contacted, only 18 (45%) responded, even after the issue of two reminders. With permission from the ENT consultant, an attempt was made to contact the rest through home visits. It was not our intention to carry out interviews at home; we had no wish to force an interview on people who had not indicated a willingness to take part. Instead, we simply attempted to find out why 22 people had failed to respond. We found that three could not be contacted, seven had moved away, two had died. Of the 10 who were contacted, eight spontaneously expressed a willingness to take part in an interview if one could be arranged, and two did not, both of whom happened to be employees of the hospital at which the study was based. Even allowing for this, the response rate is not good. This method, however, was the only one by which we could obtain a relatively unbiased population sample of people who had owned a hearing aid for a considerable amount of time. A community study was considered, but deemed to be far too costly and difficult to implement. A pilot attempt to survey private hearing aid users was extremely difficult to undertake and led us to exclude this sampling source from the study (Stevenson and Dawtrey, 1980). Finally, we rejected the suggestion that we should draw a section of the sample from lipreading classes or from clubs for the hard-of-hearing—a decision which was later vindicated when we learned that only a tiny fraction of hearing aid owners had attended lipreading classes or had even heard of clubs or societies for the hard-of-hearing.

## B. Measurement of Hearing Loss

Hearing loss was measured across the speech frequencies (0.5, 1, 2, and 4 kHz) in the better ear only. If the respondent was in doubt as to which was the better ear, thresholds were established for both ears. The audiometer used was an Amplivox 84 on loan from and calibrated by the Royal National Institute for the Deaf (RNID). Type of hearing loss was classified as *conductive, mixed,* or *sensorineural.* If the air–bone gap was 15 dB or greater across two or more frequencies, it was considered significant. Given this difference, if dB loss for bone conduction was 35 dB or less across three frequencies, the loss was classified as conductive. If greater, the loss was classified as mixed.

Speech discrimination ability was measured using phonetically balanced word lists (Boothroyd, 1968). The lists consist of 10 monosyllabic words, each containing three phonemes. Recordings of the speech lists were obtained from the RNID and played on a Ferrograph tape recorder (Type 4A). Speech was presented at 65 dB (A) output, that is, slightly above a normal conversational level. Output was from a speaker placed one metre from the respondent, who adjusted his/her hearing aid, if worn, to a comfortable listening level prior to testing. Two lists were administered, one with an aid and one without, order of presentation being alternated.

In order to obtain a subjective indicator of hearing loss, an adaptation of the scale used by Wilkins (1948) was used. Respondents were asked to place themselves at the appropriate point on the scale, both with and without a hearing aid. The self-estimate is the first item on the interview schedule (see Appendix A).

## C. Measure of Psychological Disturbance

The inventory used in the study was the SAD (States of Anxiety and Depression) which forms part of the Delusions-Symptom-Sign Inventory

(Bedford and Foulds, 1978). Before describing the SAD in detail, I would like to describe the thinking which led to the choice of the SAD as the most suitable instrument, especially in view of its central role in both studies.

The best validated and most widely used instrument for measuring and classifying psychological disturbance is probably the Present State Examination (Wing *et al.*, 1974). It is a standardised semistructured psychiatric interview which usually takes an hour or more to administer. However, the precise diagnostic categorisation which would result seemed inappropriate for a group of people, the majority of whom might exhibit no psychological abnormalities whatsoever. Furthermore, in the context of a broad-based study, it would have consumed a disproportionate amount of time.

A number of self-completion inventories are available: the Cornell Index (Weider *et al.*, 1948), the Middlesex Hospital Questionnaire, now renamed the Crown-Crisp Experiental Index (Crown and Crisp, 1979), the General Health Questionnaire (Goldberg, 1972), and the SAD section of the Delusions-Symptom-Sign Inventory (Bedford and Foulds, 1978). The disadvantages of the Cornell Index have already been discussed in relation to Mahapatra's study in the previous chapter. It is, moreover, an instrument which was developed and standardised with young male American conscripts in World War II. The Crown-Crisp Experiental Index was ruled out because it contains items which might misclassify hearing-impaired people, and because at the time, no norms were available for the general population, a shortcoming which has since been rectified (Crisp *et al.*, 1978a).

The General Health Questionnaire was, at the time of the study, the best developed and most rigorously standardised of the short inventories. The main disadvantage which precluded its use in this present study was the method of scoring used. For most questions, the respondent has to indicate degree of severity along these dimensions: "none; same as usual; more than usual; or always." The problem is that the respondent does not score unless he indicates "more than usual." This is because Goldberg is looking for evidence of recent change in psychological well-being. For a target sample that has been hearing-impaired for a number of years, the General Health Questionnaire was obviously inappropriate. Goldberg, in fact, admits that the General Health Questionnaire does not identify those with a longstanding disorder (Goldberg, 1979). Another drawback to the General Health Questionnaire, at least as far as this study is concerned, is that many items, especially the early ones, are not necessarily psychiatric in content. This is intentional on the part of the author, who wished to leave the most overtly psychiatric questions until nearer the end. However, all items score equally. It would thus be possible to reach the criterion for classification as psychiatrically disturbed on 11 of the following 15 items, out of the total of 60 in the questionnaire (Goldberg, 1972):

Been feeling perfectly well and in good health—less than usual.
Been feeling in need of a good tonic—more than usual.
Been feeling run-down and out of sorts—rather more than usual.
Felt that you are ill—rather more than usual.
Been able to concentrate on whatever you're doing—less than usual.
Been feeling mentally alert and wide awake—less alert than usual.
Been getting out of the house—less than usual.
Felt on the whole you were doing things well—less than usual.
Spent much time chatting with people—less than usual.
Been able to enjoy your normal day-to-day activities—less so than usual.
Been late getting to work or getting started with your housework—rather later than usual.
Been feeling full of energy—less energy than usual.
Been managing to keep yourself busy and occupied—rather less than usual.
Felt capable of making decisions about things—less so than usual.
Felt that you are playing a useful part in things—less useful than usual.

Goldberg has not reported an item analysis which examines the part played by items such as these. They certainly seem to indicate that the criterion for classification as disordered may not be as severe as for the Bedford and Foulds inventory, in which all the items are overtly psychiatric.

The SAD consists of 14 questions, seven on anxiety and seven on depression. It is self-administered, and takes 5–10 minutes to complete. Each question has levels of severity 0, 1, 2, and 3, resulting in a maximum possible score of $14 \times 3 = 42$. None of the items are social in nature or concerned with communication. The problem of misclassification associated with such items did not, therefore, arise. Only one item (item 9), concerned with pain in the neck or head, could possibly be considered "loaded." The contribution of item 9 to the SAD score is discussed in detail in Chapter 4.

The cut-off point recommended by the authors of the inventory is a score of 7, which is obtained or exceeded by 5% of the general population and 75% of psychiatric patients, based on 200 and 480 subjects, respectively. It is emphasised that any quantification of psychological handicap based on this screening inventory will probably be conservative, for the items are overtly psychiatric, which means that milder psychiatric symptoms may be missed. Studies using the General Health Questionnaire, for example, have found 12% of the general population to be discovered (Goldberg *et al.*, 1976), and 16% (Finlay-Jones and Burvill, 1977).

The SAD contains items on anxiety and depression only, but it fits into a hierarchical model of psychological illness described in detail by Foulds and Bedford (1975). Briefly, they have shown that people with more serious forms of disorders, such as personality disturbance and psychotic disorder, will be identified with this measure, which is at the psycho-neurotic level only. The validity of the SAD was tested against judgment of inventory items by experienced psychologists and psychiatrists as well as against psychiatric interviews.

The SAD does have a number of weaknesses, the most serious of which is that the "normal" respondents in the normative study were not given a psychiatric examination, so that information about false positives and false negatives is not available. Nor are age-related norms provided. The general population sample used by Bedford and Foulds had a mean age of 30 years (SD = 10), which was bound to be considerably younger than the hearing-impaired sample. This difference, however, should only affect results in the contra-hypothesis direction, for false positives have been found to be more common in young adults (Shepherd *et al.*, 1966; Goldberg, 1972), indicating that the norm of 5% cases in the general population may be inflated when used as a baseline for a hearing-impaired group, which is predominantly middle-aged. Finally, Goldberg, in a review of instruments similar to his own, commented that the SAD "would appear to be an instrument of acceptable validity, and is indeed in many ways comparable to the present [Goldberg's] questionnaire. Each instrument has its own advantages and limitations, and consideration of these will indicate which should be chosen for any particular research design" (Goldberg, 1972).

## D.  Suspiciousness

The following items, taken from the Paranoia Scale of the MMPI, illustrate yet again the problem of misclassification of psychologically normal people who have a hearing impairment.

No one seems to understand me.
I am sure I am being talked about.
Even when I am with people I feel lonely much of the time.
I do not often notice my ears ringing or buzzing.

Some items also tend to be rather extreme. A population which may not depart greatly from normal could well take exception to the items below (also taken from the MMPI Paranoia Scale). Such items, while possibly acceptable when interspersed throughout a personality questionnaire containing 399 items, could well seem offensive when taken together, as would have been the case had the scale been "lifted" from the MMPI.

Evil spirits possess me at times.
Someone has been trying to poison me.
I believe I am being plotted against.
I believe I am being followed.

Given the dearth of evidence for an increased incidence of paranoid mental states amongst hearing-impaired people, it was decided to use a less extreme measure, and to examine to what extent hearing-impaired people were suspicious. Campbell *et al.* (1976) have pioneered a measure of suspiciousness on a general population sample in the United States. The measure consists of the following three-part question:

a. Generally speaking, would you say that most people can be trusted, or that you can't be too careful in dealing with people?
b. Would you say that most of the time people try to be helpful, or that they are mostly just looking out for themselves?
c. Do you think that most people would try and take advantage of you if they got the chance, or would they try to be fair?

The authors of the scale report that responses to each part of the question "interrelate rather strongly" (correlations between .49 and .53). The scale, originally used in an American Quality of Life Survey, had been found to discriminate between blacks and whites, and also amongst subsamples of blacks. The authors reasoned that (Campbell *et al.*, 1976):

Black people at the lowest rung of the class ladder are least trustful of people, and trust increases among people of higher status. Black people who are divorced or separated also have high levels of distrust. . . . All of this seems to make good intuitive sense; those people who have been least successful in their encounters with society have the least reason to feel trustful of it. And this reasoning gains weight when we find that very much the same pattern we have seen amongst blacks also characterises whites [p. 455].

While no special claim is made for the measure, it does have an appealing face validity. Moreover, the items are similar to less extreme ones in the Paranoia scale of the MMPI:

Most people inwardly dislike putting themselves out to help other people.
I tend to be on guard with people who are somewhat more friendly than I expected.
Most people will use somewhat unfair means to gain profit or an advantage rather than to lose it.

The manner in which the scale was controlled on the British general population is described below.

## E. Control Groups

As the overall aim of the study was to examine the effects of hearing loss across the major life domains, sections on employment, social and family life, health, and general well-being were included. Control data were obtained from three sources. Suitable questions about work were obtained from the Multipurpose Survey (SSRC Survey Unit, 1975a), and about health and general well-being from the Quality of Life Survey (SSRC Survey Unit, 1975b). The Suspiciousness Scale was also administered in the Quality of Life Survey. Questions relating to social and family life had to be devised specifically for this study, a few adapted from a survey on psychological well-being conducted in the United States (Bradburn, 1969).

The Multipurpose Survey was carried out on a quasi-random sample of 1500 adults in the United Kingdom mainland, south of the Caledonian Canal. The Quality of Life Survey was conducted in a similar manner, except that the sample of 1000 adults was confined to urban areas. Both were undertaken by the Social Science Research Council Survey Unit, London.

The specially commissioned survey, covering social and family life, was carried out on a sample drawn from Greater London, which was matched for area of residence, age, sex, and economic activity. The size of the sample was almost exactly double that of the hearing-impaired group. It was carried out by the Social Research Division of National Opinion Polls Limited, in April, 1978. Interviewing was carried out mainly on Fridays and Saturdays in the spring of 1978. Interviewers were extensively briefed and debriefed before and after both pilot interviews and main fieldwork. A few questions from the Quality of Life Survey were also included in the National Opinion Poll (NOP) Quota Survey, where they served to orientate the respondent to the nature of the interview. A spin-off from this was that the reliability of certain items could be ascertained when subjected to different sampling and interviewing procedures.


## F. Statistical Procedures


Most data analysis was straightforward and amenable to procedures contained in the Statistical Package for the Social Sciences (Nie *et al.*, 1975). However, comparison between the hearing-impaired group and the Quality of Life and Multipurpose Surveys was much more difficult, mainly because of the massive age bias in the hearing-impaired group, thus making straightforward chi square analyses meaningless. Because of this, GLIM (General Linear Interactive Modelling) was adopted. It is a computer programme capable of multivariate analysis of contingency data (Goodman, 1970; Nelder and Wedderburn, 1972). For a detailed discussion of GLIM, see O'Muircheartaigh and Payne (1977).

Conceptually, GLIM is very simple to grasp, especially as its use is confined to categorical data. As an illustration, let us consider whether hearing-impaired people are more likely to suffer from a further physical disability than is the general population. GLIM makes it possible to control for age as well as other "nuisance" variables. In the example shown in Table 3.1, the other nuisance variable is sex, chosen because of its possible interaction with age. A straightforward comparison with the Quality of Life sample would almost certainly have provided the answer of yes, simply because hearing-impaired people are older, and the incidence of physical disability is known to increase with age.

When the data is fed into the computer, the programme yields a Grand Deviance Score (analogous to the Total Sum of Squares in an Analysis of Variance), which accounts for the main effects of survey (two levels: control and hearing-impaired), sex (two levels), age (four levels), and disability (two levels: disabled and not disabled). As well as these main effects, all possible interactions are taken into account (five two-way and four three-way). The one four-way interaction exhausts the Deviance. The Grand Deviance is reduced step by step. Firstly, the deviance due to the

TABLE 3.1

Illustration of Use of GLIM to Answer the Question: Are Hearing-impaired People More
Likely to Suffer a Further Physical Disability Than the General Population?

| Age[a] | Male | | Female | |
|---|---|---|---|---|
| | Physically disabled | Not disabled | Physically disabled | Not disabled |
| Survey 1 (Hearing-impaired group) | | | | |
| ≤39 | X[b] | X | X | X |
| 40–49 | X | X | X | X |
| 50–59 | X | X | X | X |
| 60–64 | X | X | — | — |
| Survey 2 (Quality of Life control group) | | | | |
| 39 | X | X | X | X |
| 40–49 | X | X | X | X |
| 50–59 | X | X | X | X |
| 60–64 | X | X | — | — |

[a]The age imbalance in the table is due to the exclusion of 60–64-year-old females who are postretirement age.

[b]X = number of respondents in each cell.

main effects is deducted from the Grand Deviance. The amount of Deviance which each step accounts for is virtually equivalent to a chi square
value, and can be consulted in a chi square significance table. The main
effects taken singly are of little interest, as they are design effects only. For
example, the deviance arising from the main effect of age will be extremely significant, simply because of the built-in age bias. It is by this
method, however, that the difference between the two samples due to age
alone is excluded. The other main effects of sex, survey, and disability are
similarly partialled out. We then come to the deviance resulting from the
two-way interactions. Here the important deviance is that resulting from
the interaction between physical disability and survey, which answers the
research question: What is the difference between surveys for different
levels of disability? All the other possible two-way interactions are first
obtained, thus controlling for two-way interactions amongst sex, survey,
and physical disability. Finally, the critical interaction, that between survey and disability, is computed and tested for statistical significance. Following this, any three-way interactions may be quantified in order to test
for higher order interactions, which seem conceptually plausible; in this

example, it almost could be argued that sex might interact significantly with disability differentially for hearing and hearing-impaired people.

## G. Pilot Work

The interview schedule (Appendix A) was constructed following extensive informal interviewing of hearing-impaired people, including hearing-impaired social workers studying at the Polytechnic of North London. The first version of the questionnaire was then piloted with hearing-impaired students at the Polytechnic. Research workers, social workers, audiological scientists, a psychiatrist, psychologists, sociologists, and representatives of major voluntary organisations for the hearing impaired were then consulted. The second version of the questionnaire was piloted with volunteers at an annual conference of the British Association of the Hard-of-Hearing. The third version was tested on a group of people from lipreading classes, selected by their tutors because they were believed to have social and psychological problems. The questionnaire was finalised after being piloted on a hospital sample.

Each respondent was invited by letter to attend an interview, and was specifically asked to bring his or her hearing aid, whether or not it was in use. The interview lasted between an hour and an hour and a half. It consisted of (in the order given):

a. Audiometry
b. Speech discrimination test
c. Self-evaluation of hearing loss
d. Questions concerned with onset of hearing loss; adjustment to, and benefit obtained from, the hearing aid; knowledge and use of services for hearing-impaired people.
e. Questions relating to work
f. Self-completion of the SAD
g. Questions on social and family life
h. Questions on general well-being and health.

The interviews were conducted by six interviewers—the two project directors, two research assistants, and two interviewers specifically appointed to the project. Briefing was detailed. In addition, all were trained to carry out simple audiometry by the same qualified audiometrician. Interviewing took place between November, 1976, and August, 1977.

## II. CHARACTERISTICS OF THE SAMPLE

### A.  Demographic

The age and sex distribution of the sample of 211 is given in Table 3.2. The age bias, while expected, is still rather large, even when confined to people of employment age. The mean age for men was 53 (SD=10), and for women was 48 (SD=10).

Seven (3%) of the hearing-impaired sample were separated or divorced. A GLIM analysis controlling for age and sex showed that this proportion did not differ significantly from that in the SSRC Quality of Life national survey. Moreover, the proportion in the NOP matched control group was 4.3%, which is actually higher than that for the hearing-impaired sample, though not significantly so. Therefore, there is no support for the opinion that the onset of hearing loss results in a greater likelihood of marital breakdown.

The unemployment rate for the hearing-impaired sample was 6.2%. This was found not to differ from the SSRC Multipurpose National Survey, when a GLIM analysis was carried out which controlled for age and sex. With a sample biased towards the upper age group, it is possible that unemployment might be disguised under the headings of "retired" and "permanently sick and disabled," or "housewife, full-time." A better guide to the effect of hearing impairment on employment might therefore involve a consideration of the proportion who are actually working. For the men, 83% are in employment, and for the women, 69%. Once again, a

TABLE 3.2

Age and Sex Distribution of the Sample[a]

| Sex | Age range (years) | | | | | Total |
|---|---|---|---|---|---|---|
| | 16–29 | 30–39 | 40–49 | 50–59 | 60–64 | |
| Male | 7 | 7 | 17 | 52 | 37 | 120 (57%) |
| Female | 5 | 12 | 23 | 51 | — | 91 (43%) |
| Total | 12 (6%) | 19 (9%) | 40 (19%) | 103 (49%) | 37 (17%) | 211 |

[a]If the males aged 60–64 are excluded, then the sex distribution is roughly equal.

TABLE 3.3

Social Class Distribution of the Sample Compared with the Quality of Life Survey[a]

|  | Social class | Hearing-impaired sample (%) | Quality of Life Survey (%) |
|---|---|---|---|
| I and II | Professional and intermediate | 31 | 11 |
| IIIN | Clerical | 16 | 31 |
| IIIM | Skilled manual | 33 | 25 |
| IV and V | Semiskilled and unskilled | 20 | 33 |

[a]A GLIM Analysis of Deviance which took into account the age difference showed that the hearing-impaired sample is significantly biased towards the upper social classes ($p < .001$).

GLIM analysis found that these proportions did not differ significantly from those obtained by the SSRC Multipurpose National Survey controlling for age. There is thus no support for the belief that onset of hearing loss results in a greater likelihood of unemployment.

The social class bias (Table 3.3) relates to differences within the manual and nonmanual classes. When manual is compared with nonmanual, the difference is reduced.

## B. Measures of Hearing Loss

### 1. *dB Loss*

Table 3.4 gives the distribution of dB loss. Two thirds of the sample (140) may be described as moderately impaired, with a mean loss of between 40 and 69 dB. Eleven men and two women had a profound hearing impairment. The overall mean loss was 55 dB (SD = 18); for men it was 56 dB, and for women 54 dB. The lack of a difference in mean dB loss between men and women suggests that men are not more likely to have been exposed to noise, as would have been the case if the study had been conducted in an area of heavy industry.

The mean and standard deviations for dB loss at each frequency are given in Table 3.5. The differences in mean dB loss at each frequency are highly significant statistically, but appear minimal with regard to be-

TABLE 3.4

Distribution of Hearing Loss

|  | Female | Male | Total |
|---|---|---|---|
| Mild (≤39 dB) | 12 (13%) | 22 (18%) | 34 (16%) |
| Moderate (40–69 dB) | 62 (68%) | 78 (65%) | 140 (66%) |
| Severe (70–89 dB) | 15 (17%) | 9 (8%) | 24 (12%) |
| Profound (90+ dB) | 2 (2%) | 11 (9%) | 13 (6%) |
| Total | 91 (100%) | 120 (100%) | 211 (100%) |

havioural consequences, especially in view of the large standard deviations. Despite the fact that the sample is predominantly "upper middle-aged," the dip at 4 kHz is not as marked as might be expected given the known association between high frequency loss and age. Mean dB loss was not related to age ($r = .03$).

## 2. Speech Discrimination

Speech discrimination ability was measured with and without a hearing aid. The distributions of percentage phoneme scores, both without the hearing aid and with the aid adjusted to a comfortable listening level, are given in Table 3.6. The mean unaided score was 56% (SD = 35) and aided was 79% (SD = 25).

Speech discrimination ability was not affected by sex, social class, or age. The lack of a relationship with social class is reexamined in Chapter 5, in the context of the marked relationship found in the Second Study.

TABLE 3.5

Mean dB Loss at Each Frequency Tested[a]

|  | Frequency (kHz) | | | |
|---|---|---|---|---|
|  | 0.5 | 1 | 2 | 4 |
| Mean | 49 | 51 | 55 | 63 |
| SD | 20 | 20 | 20 | 22 |
| t tests | $p < .05$ | $p < .001$ | $p < .001$ | |

[a]$N = 211$.

TABLE 3.6

Distribution of Percentage Phoneme Scores on Boothroyd's PB Word Lists[a]

| | % phonemes | | | |
| | 0–40 | 41–70 | 71–90 | 91–100 |
|---|---|---|---|---|
| Without aid | 68 (32%) | 50 (24%) | 56 (27%) | 35 (17%) |
| Aided | 17 (9%) | 29 (15%) | 77 (41%) | 65 (35%) |

[a]Twenty-three people, two of whom were not tested in the "without aid" condition, did not bring their hearing aid to the interview.

## 3. Self-estimate of Hearing Loss

A self-estimate of hearing loss was adapted from the scale used by Wilkins (1948). Respondents were asked to estimate their hearing loss with and without an aid (Table 3.7). The main purpose of the self-estimate was to obtain a subjective estimate of hearing ability to complement the objective measures of dB loss aid speech discrimination ability.

When a hearing aid is worn, only 10 people claim to have problems when facing people in a one-to-one situation (Table 3.7). It was certainly the impression of the interviewers that very few respondents experienced great problems with this kind of communication, although, of course, the interviewing conditions were near ideal, the subject matter was familiar and of obvious interest to the respondent. The figure of 10 is therefore likely to be realistic.

## 4. Relationship between Measures of Hearing Loss

Table 3.8 contains all the meaningful correlations. The highest correlations are between speech discrimination scores and mean dB loss, and are in fact almost identical to those obtained in a similar study, carried out under much more rigorous testing conditions by Tonning (1978). Correlations between self-estimate and other variables are rather low, especially those based on self-estimate when wearing a hearing aid. Whether this is due to poor validity of the self-estimate, or whether the self-estimate represents a valid measure of hearing ability independent of mean dB loss and speech discrimination test scores, is not possible to say.

TABLE 3.7

Self-estimate of Hearing Loss with and without a Hearing Aid[a]

| | Without aid | Mean dB loss | With aid | Mean dB loss |
|---|---|---|---|---|
| Can you hear a whispered voice? | 5 (2%) | 29 | 37 (18%) | 47 |
| Can you hear easily in a hall, a cinema, or a theatre? | 5 (2%) | 46 | 53 (26%) | 56 |
| Can you hear easily in a group where a few people are chatting together? | 11 (5%) | 50 | 28 (14%) | 50 |
| Can you hear easily someone facing you when they are speaking in a normal voice? | 96 (46%) | 48 | 76 (37%) | 55 |
| Can you hear easily someone facing you when they are speaking in a loud voice? | 74 (35%) | 60 | 9 (4%) | 83 |
| You cannot hear speech at all? | 20 (10%) | 78 | 1 (1%) | 98 |
| Total | 211 | | 204[b] | |

[a]Respondents are allocated to the first question on the scale to which they answer "yes."
[b]Seven people stated that they never used their hearing aid.

## 5.  Type of Hearing Loss

Audiograms were analysed to determine type of hearing loss (Table 3.9). Mean dB loss for each type of hearing loss is also given.

TABLE 3.8

Correlations between Measures of Hearing Loss

| | Mean dB loss | Unaided speech discrimination | Aided speech discrimination | Self-estimate unaided |
|---|---|---|---|---|
| Unaided speech discrimination | 0.72 | | | |
| Aided speech discrimination | 0.63 | 0.56 | | |
| Self-estimate unaided | 0.51 | 0.54 | — | |
| Self-estimate aided | 0.26 | — | 0.30 | 0.44 |

TABLE 3.9

Type of Hearing Loss

| Type of hearing loss | N | Mean dB loss |
|---|---|---|
| Sensorineural | 125 | 53 |
| Mixed | 57 | 53 |
| Conductive | 29 | 57 |

## C. Onset of Hearing Loss

In order to ascertain age of onset of hearing loss, respondents were asked, "How old were you when you first had trouble with your hearing?"

As Table 3.10 shows, half of the new patients who had apparently obtained their first aid between 1 and 6 years beforehand, had in fact had problems with hearing for considerably longer. Of the 182 respondents aged 40 or over, 35 (19%) had actually first experienced hearing problems while still at school.

It became apparent, while interviewing was taking place at the first hearing aid clinic, that a number of respondents had previously obtained an aid privately or from another hearing aid clinic. For the second two hospitals, the questionnaire was amended slightly so that respondents were additionally asked at what age they had acquired a hearing aid, from whatever source. For the two clinics at which these data were collected, the mean duration between onset of hearing problems and acquisition of an aid was 13.2 years ($N = 131$).

One would expect the number of years estimated to have elapsed between onset and acquisition of an aid to tally reasonably well with the

TABLE 3.10

Onset of Hearing Loss

| Age at interview (years) | N | Age of onset (years) | Percentage (%) |
|---|---|---|---|
| 16–39 | 29 | 16 | 51 (51 out of 29) |
| 40–49 | 40 | 30 | 52 (21 out of 40) |
| 50–64 | 142 | 40 | 45 (64 out of 142) |

TABLE 3.11

Comparison of Two Questions Related to Onset of Hearing Loss[a]

| Amount of time elapsed between realisation of hearing difficulty and visit to general practitioner | Mean number of years between onset of hearing difficulty and acquisition of a hearing aid |
| --- | --- |
| ≤6 months | 11.2 years ($N = 51$) |
| 7 months–3 years | 9.4 years ($N = 44$) |
| >3 years | 20.5 years ($N = 36$) |

[a]These figures are based on two hearing aid clinics only, for reasons explained in the text.

amount of time elapsed between first awareness of hearing loss and contact with the general practitioner. As Table 3.11 shows, this was not the case. It appears, therefore, that subjective estimates relating to the onset or course of hearing loss are very unreliable. An audiological physician has commented on similar difficulties, even based on rigorous history taking (Stephens, 1982). The only possible conclusion is that a large proportion of hearing-impaired people wait a considerable number of years before they seek advice.

A study of visual handicap suggests that a considerable time lapse between onset and referral may be a common feature of many handicapping conditions, especially where deterioration is gradual. Abel (1976) reported the length of time between onset of visual handicap and date of registration as blind or partially sighted for 103 respondents, aged 40–64, as:

| | |
| --- | --- |
| <3 years | 36 (35%) |
| 3–9 years, 11 months | 24 (23%) |
| 10+ years | 43 (42%) |

## D. Progression of Hearing Loss

Progression of hearing loss was measured by comparing our audiograms with those provided by two out of the three hospitals. As Table 3.12 shows there was little overall deterioration in the two hospitals for which comparison was possible ($N = 167$). The mean drop of 5 dB in hearing level could largely be accounted for in terms of difference in quality of testing

TABLE 3.12

Progression of Hearing Loss

| Hospital | N | Hospital audiogram[a] | First study | r |
|---|---|---|---|---|
| No. 1 | 78 | 46 dB (SD = 16) | 51 dB (SD = 15) | .72 |
| No. 2 | 89 | 54 dB (SD = 17) | 58 dB (SD = 18) | .78 |
| Total | 167 | 50 dB (SD = 17) | 55 dB (SD = 17) | .76 |

[a] 1 to 7 years previously.

conditions between audiometric booths and the reasonably quiet rooms in which our testing took place. Two respondents experienced a marked improvement in hearing level (15 + dB) while 13 (8%) had suffered a marked deterioration. There was no systematic variation within the time interval between the two sets of audiograms.

## E. The Hearing Aid

One hundred respondents possessed a postaural hearing aid and 111, a bodyworn one. As expected, people with postaural hearing aids use them a great deal more (Table 3.13). The table also shows the relationship between use and degree of hearing loss. While the trend is in the predicted direction, the differences are by no means large.

Another approach to the measurement of hearing aid benefit was to use speech discrimination gain scores (Thomas & Gilhome Herbst, 1980a). Of the 189 respondents who were tested in both the unaided and aided conditions, 21 heard worse with an aid than without, 20 obtained no increment in their ability to discriminate speech when wearing an aid, and 38 obtained an increment of 10% or less phoneme discrimination ability with an aid (based on a maximum score of 83% in the unaided condition). Thus, 69 (42%) of those who brought their aid to the interview appeared not to benefit or to benefit little from its use. This finding has been confirmed by Haggard et al. (1981b). There was a tendency, as might be expected, for those who obtained little or no benefit from the hearing aid to make less use of it. The tendency was not marked, however, indicating that certain people may persevere with aids from which they obtain little benefit.

TABLE 3.13

Hearing Aid Type by Hearing Aid Usage by Mean dB Loss

| Aid | Amount of time worn | | | | | Mean dB Loss |
|---|---|---|---|---|---|---|
| | Always | Often | Sometimes | Rarely | Never | |
| Bodyworn ($N = 98$) | 10% | 17% | 21% | 16% | 35% | 59 dB |
| Postaural ($N = 111$) | 38% | 21% | 25% | 12% | 5% | 51 dB |
| Mean dB loss | 64 dB | 53 dB | 52 dB | 51 dB | 49 dB | 55 dB |

It is generally accepted that amplification is sufficient to overcome conductive, but not sensorineural, hearing loss (Noble, 1978). The relationship between type of hearing loss and speech discrimination ability, however, has only been investigated under laboratory conditions. It has been demonstrated, for example, that increasing amplification will eventually result in 100% discrimination for people with conductive losses; for those with sensorineural losses, the relationship between amplification and speech discrimination ability follows an inverted U-curve, the plateau mostly occurring well below 100% discrimination (Hood and Poole, 1971). It is important, therefore, that type of hearing loss should be taken into account in any attempt to measure hearing aid benefit based on the difference between unaided and aided speech discrimination. A one-way Analysis of Covariance of speech discrimination gain scores was carried out with type of hearing loss as the independent variable, and mean dB loss as the covariate (Table 3.14A). Table 3.14B contains the means for each type of loss, both unadjusted and adjusted, to take account of the covariate of mean dB loss. As expected, those with conductive losses make very much greater gains between unaided and aided speech discrimination. Those with conductive losses perform significantly worse in the unaided condition and significantly better in the aided condition. Performance of those with mixed and sensorineural losses do not differ significantly.

A number of more complicated analyses were undertaken in order to quantify the effect of age, sex, type of aid worn, and amount of time that the aid was worn. None of these variables was found to affect the relationship between type of loss and speech discrimination scores, either singly or interactively. Type of hearing loss is therefore an important factor in speech discrimination ability, and as expected, those with conductive

TABLE 3.14A

Analysis of Covariance of Speech Discrimination Gain Scores[a]

| Source | df | sos | ms | F | p |
|---|---|---|---|---|---|
| Type of hearing loss | 2 | 11,153 | 5,576 | 7.7 | .001 |
| Mean dB loss (covariate) | 1 | 12,610 | 12,610 | 17.4 | .001 |
| Residual | 183 | 132,521 | 724 | | |
| Totals | 186 | 157,212 | | | |

[a]$N = 187$.

TABLE 3.14B

Mean Speech Discrimination Scores (Percentage of Phonemes) by Type of Hearing Loss

| Type of loss (N) | Unadjusted means | | Adjusted means[a] | | |
|---|---|---|---|---|---|
| | Unaided (SD) | Aided (SD) | Unaided | Aided | Gain |
| Conductive (28) | 40 (37.1) | 85 (20.9) | 43 | 85 | 42 |
| Mixed (51) | 56 (33.4) | 82 (20.4) | 58 | 83 | 25 |
| Sensorineural (108) | 58 (34.1) | 76 (27.3) | 55 | 75 | 20 |

[a]Adjusted to take into account the effect of the covariate of mean dB loss.

losses gain more from using a hearing aid than do those with sensorineural losses. Much of the difference, however, is attributable to a significantly poorer performance by those with conductive losses in the unaided condition. Respondents with conductive losses do not attain 100% discrimination as they do under laboratory conditions, and although they perform significantly better than respondents with sensorineural losses, the difference is not very marked. Those with sensorineural losses do not, in general, appear to gain very much from wearing an aid. For further details, see Thomas and Gilhome Herbst (1981).

# CHAPTER FOUR

## *Psychological and Psychosocial Effects*

### I. PSYCHOLOGICAL DISTURBANCE

Out of the sample of 211 hearing-impaired adults of employment age, 205 completed the SAD, a subsection of the Delusions-Symptom-Sign Inventory, which consists of the scales of anxiety and depression (Bedford and Foulds, 1978). Of the six who did not complete the inventory, four were unable to and two refused. A summary distribution of scores, which includes a comparison with normative data, is given in Table 4.1, classified according to Bedford and Foulds's suggestions; thus, a score of 0–2 indicates normality, a score of 3–6 is intermediate, and a score of 7+ indicates psychological disturbance. It will be noted that 19% may be described as disturbed, with a further 20% in the intermediate category.

The separate scales of anxiety and depression were found to intercorrelate highly: $r = 0.70$. This compares with an intercorrelation of 0.69 in the normative study. The correlations between the anxiety and depression scores and the overall SAD score were 0.92 and 0.93. The scales are obviously not independent, and the SAD will therefore be treated as a screening device and not a diagnostic one.

### A. Demographic Factors

The proportion of psychologically disturbed patients, by age and by sex, is given in Table 4.2. Unfortunately, Bedford and Foulds do not provide

TABLE 4.1

TABLE 4.1

Frequency Distribution of Scores on the SAD

| SAD score | General population (%) | Psychiatric patients (%) | Hearing-impaired respondents[a] (%) |
|-----------|------------------------|--------------------------|--------------------------------------|
| 0–2       | 81                     | 12                       | 61 ($N = 125$)                       |
| 3–6       | 14                     | 14                       | 20 ($N = 41$)                        |
| 7+        | 5                      | 75                       | 19 ($N = 39$)                        |

[a]The proportion screened disturbed in the hearing-impaired sample with a score of 7+ differed significantly from the general population ($p < .001$).

age-related normative data, other than to give the mean age of the normal sample as 30.4 (SD = 10.2). This might make comparison difficult, because two thirds of the normative sample are probably between 20 and 40, while two thirds of the hearing-impaired sample are known to be over 50. However, Shepherd *et al.* (1966) found the proportion of people psychologically disturbed in a general practice study to be fairly constant within the 25- to 65-year age range. Similarly, Goldberg (1972) found no relationship between psychological disturbance and age in a major normative study of 553 adults between the ages of 15 and 74. The age bias in the hearing-impaired sample should not, therefore, prejudice comparison with norms based on a younger age group. The larger proportion of females found to be psychologically disturbed is in accord with almost all general population studies.

It will be recalled that there is a highly significant social class bias towards the upper social classes in the hearing-impaired sample. However, most general population studies have found that psychological disturbance

TABLE 4.2

Proportion of Psychologically Disturbed Respondents by Age and by Sex

| Age | Sex | |
|-----|-----|-----|
|     | Male | Female |
| 16–29 | 50% (3 out of 6) | 40% (2 out of 5) |
| 30–59 | 12% (9 out of 73) | 24% (20 out of 84) |
| 60–64 | 14% (5 out of 37) | |

is greater in the lower social classes (e.g., Crisp *et al.,* 1978b; Goldberg, 1972). Therefore, any bias resulting from the social class structure in the hearing-impaired sample is unlikely to result in an overestimate of psychological disturbance. In the hearing-impaired sample, there was no apparent relationship between social class and psychological disturbance—20% in social classes I through IIIN and 22% in social classes IIIM through V were found to be psychologically disturbed.

Overall, it appears highly unlikely that the demographic biases in the hearing-impaired sample affect the proportion of respondents identified as psychologically disturbed. There are a number of reasons for believing that the proportion identified as psychologically disturbed in the hearing-impaired sample may be an underestimate of the true extent of disturbance. Firstly, the SAD, in common with similar inventories, stresses recency of signs and symptoms, thus possibly missing people with longstanding disorders. Secondly, at one of the hearing aid clinics from which the sample was drawn, the senior ENT consultant believed that patients already known to have social and psychological problems should not be interviewed by nonmedical personnel. They were thus excluded from the sample lists which the hearing aid clinic provided for the study. Thirdly, the SAD (as discussed in Chapter 3) appears more overtly psychiatric than its sister inventories. Goldberg's General Health Questionnaire, for example, has been shown to identify 16% in a community prevalence study in Australia (Finlay-Jones and Burvill, 1977) and 12% in this country (Goldberg *et al.,* 1976), compared with 5% for the SAD.

On the other hand, people visitng their general practitioners or attending hospital outpatient departments are known to be more psychologically disturbed than the general population (Goldberg *et al.,* 1976). However, most of the hearing-impaired sample had ceased to be "patients" in the usual sense, contact with the hearing aid clinics being maintained for practical (rather than medical) reasons, for replacement and repair of aids, and for the issue of batteries.

## B. Item Analysis

A serious drawback to many psychological inventories concerns the likelihood of misclassification of hearing-impaired people who are psychologically normal (see Chapter 3). Before the main fieldwork stage was carried out, both professional and lay people were asked if they thought that any of the items of the SAD might contribute to a misclassification. The only item mentioned was number 9: "Recently, I have had a pain or tense feeling in my neck or head." The opinion expressed was that hearing-impaired individuals would be more likely than the normally hearing to suffer head pains which were not psychosomatic in origin. In order to examine the effect of this item on the scale, it is necessary to understand the scoring system used for the SAD. In all there are 14 questions, and each question has four levels of severity: 0, 1, 2, and 3. A score of 0 indicates that the symptom is not present. Each item which is then agreed upon is further graded for severity from 1 to 3, with 3 being the most severe. Thus, the maximum score is $14 \times 3 = 42$. It will be recalled that the cut-off score is 7. Table 4.3 illustrates that item 9 figures prominently, and it is agreed to the same extent as is item 5: "Recently, I have been depressed without knowing why."

When the 39 respondents screened as psychologically disturbed were treated as a separate subsample, item 9 did not figure as prominently (Table 4.4), contributing less than item 5 to the overall score, and roughly the same as items 1, 4, and 10.

More to the point, an attempt was made to see what would happen if

TABLE 4.3

Frequency Distribution of Individuals Items Scores for the SAD

| Degree of severity | Item number | | | | | | | | | | | | | |
|---|---|---|---|---|---|---|---|---|---|---|---|---|---|---|
| | 1 | 2 | 3 | 4 | 5[a] | 6 | 7 | 8 | 9[a] | 10 | 11 | 12 | 13 | 14 |
| 1 (least severe) | 34 | 20 | 29 | 28 | 47 | 10 | 20 | 23 | 48 | 21 | 34 | 9 | 20 | 9 |
| 2 (moderately severe) | 15 | 10 | 5 | 11 | 12 | 4 | 10 | 10 | 16 | 10 | 13 | 13 | 7 | 4 |
| 3 (most severe) | 3 | 0 | 2 | 3 | 6 | 0 | 0 | 2 | 3 | 6 | 1 | 1 | 2 | 2 |
| Total[b] | 73 | 40 | 45 | 59 | 89 | 18 | 40 | 49 | 89 | 59 | 63 | 38 | 40 | 23 |

[a]Item 5 is concerned with depression, and item 9 with head pains (see text).
[b]Totals are weighted; for example, for item 1, the total of 73 is made up of $34 \times 1$, $+ 15 \times 2$, $+ 3 \times 3$.

TABLE 4.4

Frequency Distribution of Individual Item scores of 7+ for the SAD ($N = 39$)

| Degree of severity | Item number | | | | | | | | | | | | | |
| --- | --- | --- | --- | --- | --- | --- | --- | --- | --- | --- | --- | --- | --- | --- |
| | 1 | 2 | 3 | 4 | 5 | 6 | 7 | 8 | 9 | 10 | 11 | 12 | 13 | 14 |
| 1 (least) | 14 | 12 | 13 | 10 | 18 | 9 | 14 | 12 | 14 | 7 | 10 | 3 | 13 | 9 |
| 2 | 11 | 9 | 5 | 9 | 9 | 4 | 10 | 8 | 9 | 9 | 9 | 13 | 7 | 4 |
| 3 (most) | 2 | 0 | 3 | 5 | 0 | 0 | 2 | 3 | 6 | 1 | 1 | 1 | 2 | 2 |
| Total | 42 | 30 | 29 | 37 | 51 | 17 | 34 | 34 | 41 | 41 | 31 | 32 | 29 | 23 |

item 9 were excluded for those who were psychologically disturbed. However, if an item is taken out, then it will presumably influence the cut-off score. Because of this, the criterion for classification as psychologically disturbed was reduced by the least possible amount, by 1 point to 6. As a result, 4 respondents now entered the normal category. However, a further two respondents, originally screened as normal, had now become "abnormal," with a score of 6, which did not include a contribution from item 9. The net loss, therefore, would have been 2. Exactly the same result could have been obtained had item 5 (on depression) been excluded. The exclusion of item 9, therefore, would have had virtually no effect on the proportion identified as psychologically disturbed.

## C. Effect of Other Disabilities on the SAD

In the Quality of Life Survey administered to the national sample of the general population, the following question was asked: "Do you yourself have any longstanding physical disability or health trouble?" The hearing-impaired sample was asked the same question, except that participants were instructed to exclude hearing impairment. The GLIM[1] analysis is summarised in Table 4.5. As might be expected, there is a significant interaction between age and physical disability. In other words, as respondents get older, they are more likely to suffer further physical dis-

[1]All GLIM analyses are presented in summary form. For full details, see Morgan (1978).

TABLE 4.5

GLIM Analysis of Differences in Presence of Physical Disability or Health Trouble between the Hearing-Impaired Sample and the Quality of Life General Population Sample

| Interaction effects | df | Deviance ($\chi^2$) | Significance[a] |
|---|---|---|---|
| Sex/physical disability or health trouble | 2 | 3.9 | NS |
| Age/physical disability or health trouble | 6 | 73.91 | .001 |
| Survey/physical disability or health trouble | 2 | 25.13 | .001 |

[a]The higher order three-way interactions were all insignificant. NS, Not significant.

ability or health trouble, Even after this has been controlled, there is still a highly significant interaction between survey (Quality of Life Survey and Survey of Hearing Impaired) and physical disability or health trouble (present or absent). Thus, the hearing impaired are more likely to suffer a second disability or health trouble (over and above that of hearing impairment) than the general population is to suffer a first one. Given this difference, it was now important to investigate to what extent the second disability or health trouble was implicated in psychological disturbance, given the likely effect of physical disability or health trouble on psychological well-being.

In the GLIM analysis in Table 4.6, a self-estimate of visual ability was also taken into account. All the two-way and three-way interactions that include the SAD score are given. It is obvious that the only interaction

TABLE 4.6

GLIM Analysis of Physical Disability (two levels), SAD Score (three levels), Mean dB Loss (three levels), and Eyesight (two levels)

| Effects | df | Deviance ($\chi^2$) | Significance[a] |
|---|---|---|---|
| SAD/physical disability | 1 | .08 | NS |
| SAD/eyesight | 1 | 2.12 | NS |
| SAD/mean dB loss | 2 | 11.04 | .01 |
| SAD/mean dB loss/eyesight | 2 | .34 | NS |
| SAD/physical disability/eyesight | 1 | 3.09 | NS |
| SAD/physical disability/mean dB loss | 2 | .03 | NS |

[a]NS, Not significant.

which stands out is that between the SAD and mean dB loss. Furthermore, this interaction appears to exhaust the deviance in that the three-way interactions were insignificant. It seems fair to conclude that psychological disturbance is related to hearing loss and not to any other form of physical disability or health trouble.


## D. The SAD, General Well-being, and Stress


Table 4.7 shows how the answers differed between the normal section of the sample ($N = 166$), and those identified as psychologically disturbed ($N = 39$) with regard to discrete questions in the interview schedule covering general psychological well-being. In a similar vein, Table 4.8 compares the responses of the disturbed and normal sections of the sample with regard to indicators of stress in the everyday life domains covered in the questionnaire. It is clear that the SAD score is closely related to indicators of stress in the major life domains, to general psychological well-being variables, and perhaps more importantly, to everyday life domains.

To summarise so far, the proportion of the hearing-impaired sample identified as psychologically disturbed is roughly four times as high as that found in the general population. Demographic biases in the sample do not account for the increased incidence of psychological disturbance. On the contrary, there are a number of reasons for believing it to be an underesti-

TABLE 4.7

Relationship between SAD and Discrete Questions Related to Psychological Well-being

| Question | Normal section of sample (%) | SAD cases[a] (%) |
|---|---|---|
| Worry about being near to a nervous breakdown? | 8 (13 out of 166) | 46 (18 out of 39) |
| Consulted a doctor about a nervous problem? | 30 (49 out of 166) | 61 (23 out of 38) |
| Worry "a great deal" in general? | 41 (63 out of 155) | 84 (32 out of 39) |
| Trouble getting to sleep? | 10 (16 out of 165) | 41 (16 out of 39) |
| Trouble staying asleep? | 13 (21 out of 163) | 33 (13 out of 39) |

[a]In all cases, $p < .01$.

TABLE 4.8

Relationship between SAD and Stress in Everyday Life Domains

| Domain | Question | Normal section of sample (%) | SAD cases[a] (%) |
|---|---|---|---|
| Health | Dissatisfaction with state of health? | 30 (49 out of 166) | 69 (27 out of 39) |
| Social | No friends? | 1 (2 out of 165) | 24 (9 out of 38) |
| Family | Hearing loss adversely affects marriage? | 20 (26 out of 130) | 60 (15 out of 25) |
| Work | Hearing loss affects work? | 13 (17 out of 133) | 42 (11 out of 26) |
| At interview | (Rated by interviewer as upset) | 10 (16 out of 164) | 31 (11 out of 39) |

[a]In all cases, $p < .01$.

mate. An item in the SAD which could have contributed to misclassification was found not to have done so. Other physical disabilities were not related to the SAD. Finally, the SAD was validated by its relationship with other measures of stress and psychological well-being.

## II. PSYCHOLOGICAL DISTURBANCE, MEAN dB LOSS, AND SPEECH DISCRIMINATION

Table 4.9 describes the relationship between dB loss and psychological disturbance measured by the SAD. For those with a mean loss of 70 dB or greater, the likelihood of being psychologically disturbed increases substantially. An Analysis of Variance of mean dB loss revealed that the SAD was a significant main factor, controlling for age, sex, and social class. As might be expected, an analysis confined to those with a mean hearing loss of less than 70 dB revealed no effect whatsoever due to the SAD.

The SAD was also a significant factor in an Analysis of Variance of aided speech discrimination scores. The effect disappeared, however, when the covariate of mean dB loss was introduced into the analysis. The level of significance of the effect of the SAD on aided speech discrimination ($p < .15$) suggested there might be an effect related to a subsample, such as those in Table 4.10 who are poor discriminators.

TABLE 4.9

Relationship between Mean dB Loss and the SAD

| Result of SAD | Mean dB loss | | | |
|---|---|---|---|---|
| | (norm) | 49 (mild) | 50–69 (moderate) | 70+ (severe)[a] |
| Normal | 380 | 72 | 75 | 19 |
| SAD cases | 20 | 14 | 12 | 13 |
| Total | 400 | 86 | 87 | 32 |
| % SAD | 5% | 17% | 14% | 41% |

[a]The proportion of SAD cases with a severe pure tone loss differed significantly from those with mild and moderate losses taken together ($p < .001$).

In order to measure the combined effect of a severe pure tone loss and poor speech discrimination on the SAD, the 32 people with a mean dB loss of 70 or more were examined. Of the entire 32, 9 who appeared to have a surprisingly good speech discrimination score of more than 70% phonemes correct were then excluded. The 23 left had a severe loss combined with a poor speech discrimination score, even when wearing a hearing aid. Of these, two were illiterate and did not complete the inventory. The results for the other 21 are given in Table 4.11, together with the comparison

TABLE 4.10

Relationship between Aided Speech Discrimination Ability and the SAD

| Result of SAD | Speech discrimination ability (aided) | | |
|---|---|---|---|
| | Good (91–100% phonemes correct) | Fair (71–90% phonemes correct) | Poor[a] (≤70% phonemes correct) |
| Normal | 54 | 63 | 31 |
| SAD cases | 9 | 13 | 13 |
| Total | 63 | 76 | 44 |
| % SAD cases (norm = 5%) | 14% | 17% | 30% |

[a]The proportion of poor discriminators who were SAD cases differed significantly from the other two proportions taken together ($p < .05$).

TABLE 4.11

Effect of Combining Measures of dB Loss and Aided Speech Discrimination Ability on the SAD

| Result of SAD | Mean dB loss <70 dB and speech discrimination ability >70% | Mean dB loss ≥70 dB and speech discrimination ability ≤ 70% |
|---|---|---|
| Normal | 109 | 9 |
| SAD cases | 20 | 12 |
| Totals | 129 | 21 |
| % SAD cases | 16% | 57% |
| (norm = 5%) | $p < .01$ | |

group of people with a moderate mean dB loss and good aided speech discrimination.

The proportion of psychological disturbance increases dramatically for those who have a severe dB loss compounded by poor speech discrimination ability. It is understandable that those who appear able to compensate for severe pure tone losses with reasonable speech discrimination scores may not be disordered. Not included in Table 4.11 are those with poor speech discrimination scores, although they only have mild or moderate hearing losses. There were 35 such cases, only 3 (9%) of whom were psychologically disturbed, a finding which is puzzling and difficult to interpret. However, the relationship between severe hearing loss (a mean loss of 70 dB or more and a speech discrimination score of 70% or less) and the SAD score still stands, and was confirmed by a two-way Analysis of Variance of aided speech discrimination scores with the SAD and degree of hearing loss as the main factors. The interaction between dB loss and the SAD was significant ($p < .05$). The breakdown of the relationship quantified in the two-way Analysis of Variance is given in Table 4.12.

In order to be absolutely sure, a repeat Analysis of Variance confined to those with a hearing loss of less than 70 dB was carried out. In this analysis, the SAD factor lost its significance, as did the two-way interaction between degree of hearing loss and the SAD. It is clear, therefore, that the interaction effect between SAD and the mean dB loss is due to the subsample of cases with a hearing loss of 70 dB or greater. In other words,

TABLE 4.12

Breakdown of Aided Speech Discrimination Scores by Degree of Hearing Loss and
Psychological Disturbance[a]

| Psychological disturbance | Mean dB loss | | | | |
|---|---|---|---|---|---|
| | ≤39 | 40–49 | 50–59 | 60–69 | 70+ |
| Normal | 91 | 90 | 81 | 77 | 62 |
| SAD cases | 88 | 91 | 85 | 74 | 36 |

[a]The variable averaged is the percentage speech discrimination score when wearing a hearing aid.

those who have a severe hearing loss and in addition are poorly able to discriminate speech are far more likely to be psychologically disturbed. This is one of the major findings of the First Study, first described by Thomas and Gilhome Herbst (1980b). The characteristics of this severely hearing-impaired subsample are described later on in this chapter.

## III. PSYCHOLOGICAL DISTURBANCE AND OTHER HEARING LOSS VARIABLES

Sensorineural hearing loss is commonly associated with sound distortion and side effects such as vertigo and recruitment. It is, therefore, reasonable to expect that it will result in greater stress than will conductive hearing loss, which simply attenuates (rather than distorts) sound, and should therefore be more easily compensated by hearing aid amplification. Nevertheless, both conductive and sensorineural hearing loss appear equally stressful (Table 4.13).

In all, 89 respondents suffered tinnitus, 17 (19%) of whom were identified by the SAD, the same proportion as for the sample overall. While it is obviously stressful to be subjected to "noises in the head," it does not seem that such stress leads to psychological disturbance. Severity of tinnitus might be related to psychological disturbance, but no attempt was made to quantify this variable.

As Table 4.14 illustrates, there is no apparent relationship between time

TABLE 4.13

Relationship between Type of Hearing Loss and the SAD[a]

| | Type of hearing loss | | |
| Result of SAD | Sensorineural | Mixed | Conductive |
|---|---|---|---|
| Normal | 101 | 42 | 22 |
| SAD cases | 22 | 10 | 7 |
| Total | 123 | 51 | 29 |
| % SAD cases | 18% | 20% | 24% |

[a]All differences NS.

of onset of hearing loss and the SAD. Duration of hearing loss is a very crude measure of onset in that some respondents who had been affected for 20 years, for example, will have had a hearing loss since childhood, while others who have been affected for 20 years may not have suffered onset until they were in their 30s or 40s. This may explain why there is no discernible pattern distinguishing the psychologically disturbed from the rest of the sample, it being difficult to believe that the time elapsed since onset of hearing loss is unimportant for psychological well-being.

Table 4.15A shows that, though not significant, there may be a relationship between self-estimate of hearing impairment and the SAD. As Table 4.15B shows, however, any such relationship does not derive from any independence of the self-estimate from other measures of hearing impairment, but from the relationship between the self-estimate and dB loss. This is to be expected, given that the only sizable correlation between

TABLE 4.14

Relationship between Years of Trouble with Hearing and the SAD[a]

| Years of trouble with hearing | N | Number of SAD cases | Percentage of SAD cases (%) |
|---|---|---|---|
| 0–10 | 73 | 14 | 19 |
| 11–30 | 79 | 17 | 22 |
| 31+ | 48 | 8 | 17 |

[a]All differences NS.

TABLE 4.15A

Relationship between Self-estimate of Hearing Loss and the SAD

| | Without hearing aid[a] | | With hearing aid[b] | |
|---|---|---|---|---|
| Result of SAD | Categories 1–4 (lesser impairment) | Categories 5–6 (greater impairment) | Categories 1–3 (less impairment) | Categories 4–5 (greater impairment) |
| Normal | 99 | 67 | 100 | 62 |
| SAD cases | 18 | 21 | 17 | 19 |
| Total | 117 | 88 | 117 | 81 |
| % SAD cases | 15% | 24% | 15% | 23% |

[a]$\chi^2 = 2.43$; NS.
[b]$\chi^2 = 2.56$; NS.

TABLE 4.15B

Breakdown of Relationship between Self-estimate of Hearing Loss and the SAD,
Controlling for Mean dB Loss

| | Without an aid | | | With an aid | | |
|---|---|---|---|---|---|---|
| Self-estimate | $N$ | SAD cases[a] | Mean loss[b] | $N$ | SAD cases[a] | Mean loss[b] |
| Can hear whisper | 5 | 1 (20%) | 29 dB | 36 | 3 (8%) | 47 dB |
| Can hear in hall | 5 | 0 (0%) | 46 dB | 53 | 10 (19%) | 56 dB |
| Can hear in group | | | | | | |
| Can hear normal voice | 11 | 2 (18%) | 50 dB | 28 | 4 (14%) | 50 dB |
| face-to-face | 96 | 15 (16%) | 48 dB | 73 | 15 (21%) | 53 dB |
| Can hear loud voice face-to-face | 71 | 14 (20%) | 59 dB | 8 | 4 (50%) | 84 dB |
| Cannot hear speech | 17 | 7 (41%) | 78 dB | — | — | — |

[a]Overall % of SAD cases = 19%.
[b]Mean dB loss = 54 dB.

the self-estimate and other measures of hearing impairment was that between self-estimates and dB loss.

Hearing aid benefit was measured by amount of time the hearing aid was
worn, and also by gain scores between unaided and aided speech discrimination. In neither case was there a relationship between hearing aid benefit
and the SAD. Wearing a hearing aid does not, of itself, appear to reduce
stress associated with hearing loss, although speech discrimination ability,
which presumably is mediated at least partly by hearing aid usage, is
related to psychological disturbance.

## IV. SUSPICIOUSNESS

Responses to the Suspiciousness Scale are given in Table 4.16. The
questions were controlled on the Quality of Life Survey (SSRC Survey
Unit, 1975b). A GLIM analysis taking age and sex into account revealed
no differences, nor even any hint of a difference, between the hearing
impaired and general population samples. It is extremely unlikely that the
answers to these questions were the result of any systematic "response
set," because health and well-being questions asked just prior to the ones
on suspicion were found to yield statistically significant differences when
compared with the general population. After treating each question separately and finding no differences, those who had answered all three ques-

TABLE 4.16

Responses to Items on Suspiciousness Scale

| Item | Agree | Disagree |
|------|-------|----------|
| Generally speaking, would you say that most people can be trusted, or that you can't be too careful in dealing with people? | 106 (52%) | 98 (48%) |
| Would you say that most of the time people try to be helpful, or that generally they are just looking out for themselves? | 126 (61%) | 80 (39%) |
| Do you think that most people would try to take advantage of you if they got the chance, or would they try to be fair? | 73 (36%) | 131 (64%) |

tions in the suspicious direction were examined. Amongst the hearing impaired, 34 (17%) fell into this category. This proportion was exactly the same as that in the Quality of Life sample. The direct comparison is possible because the GLIM analyses of individual items revealed that the possible nuisance variables of age and sex had no effect.

In Chapter 2, the supposed relationship between hearing loss and paranoid mental states was found to be unsubstantiated. Now it seems that hearing-impaired individuals are not even mildly suspicious.

## V.  HEALTH AND GENERAL WELL-BEING

It is clear from Table 4.17A that hearing loss has an adverse effect on general state of health. In Table 4.17B, it can be seen that three out of the six items were also asked of the NOP matched control group. It will be recalled that the purpose of using this control group was to obtain data on family and social life, and that these three items were presented to the NOP control group at the beginning of the interview in order to create a suitable ambience. It is obvious that the significant differences found between the

TABLE 4.17

| A. Difference on Health Items between Quality of Life and Hearing-impaired samples (GLIM) | | B. Difference between NOP Matched Control Group and Hearing-Impaired Sample on Three of the Items | |
|---|---|---|---|
| Item | $p$ | Hearing-impaired group | NOP control group |
| Getting to sleep | NS[a] | | |
| Staying asleep | .005 | | |
| Overall satisfaction with state of health | .001 | | |
| Suffering a further disability or health trouble | .01 | 28% (58 out of 208) | 13% (55 out of 418) $p < .001$ |
| Not having enough energy for day-to-day activities | .01 | 48% (100 out of 207) | 17% (114 out of 418) $p < .01$ |
| Consulting a doctor or anyone else concerning a nervous problem | .005 | 36% (75 out of 207) | 27% (112 out of 418) $p < .02$ |

[a]NS, Not significant.

hearing-impaired sample and the Quality of Life sample also applied when the hearing-impaired group was compared with the NOP matched control group, thereby validating the use of the Quality of Life Survey for control purposes.

## VI. EMPLOYMENT, SOCIAL AND FAMILY LIFE

### A. Employment

The onset of hearing loss does not result in an increased likelihood of unemployment. Nor, apparently, is it associated with "underemployment," that is, being forced into a job with diminished status, or lessened promotion prospects. It also seems that hearing-impaired people do not see themselves as being forced to change jobs in the future. These findings are confirmed by Hyde *et al.* (1981) in a study carried out in Australia. As Hyde and his associates point out, such findings are "in contrast to the official statement of the British Society of Audiology (Markides *et al.*, 1979), which lists a range of severe vocational limitations including difficulty in maintaining employment, in promotion, in changes of employment, underemployment, and social restrictions at work."

On the other hand, respondents were more prone to worry about work, and were less happy at work than were their hearing counterparts (Table 4.18A). Those items which would not be controlled on the general popula-

TABLE 4.18A

Comparison between the Hearing Impaired and Multipurpose Survey
Control Group on Questions Relating to Employment (GLIM)

| Item | Level of significance[b] |
|------|------------------------|
| Proportion unemployed | NS |
| Present job right for abilities | NS |
| Likelihood of promotion | NS |
| Likelihood of changing jobs in the future | NS |
| Unhappy at work | $p < .01$ |
| Worry about work[a] | $p < .025$ |

[a]The last item, concerning worry about work, is based on a comparison with the Quality of Life Survey.

[b]NS, Not significant.

TABLE 4.18B

Relationship between Psychological Disturbance and Well-being at Work

| Question | Section of sample | | $p$ |
|---|---|---|---|
| | Normal | SAD cases | |
| Changed jobs due to hearing loss? | 14% (19 out of 140) | 37% (7 out of 19) | .01 |
| Hearing loss affects work a lot? | 13% (17 out of 133) | 42% (11 out of 26) | .01 |

tion because of reference to hearing loss were examined for their relationship with the SAD (Table 4.18B), and confirm that work is likely to prove a source of stress for hearing-impaired people.

## B.  Social Life

In comparison with the NOP matched control group, the hearing-impaired group was found to be more lonely, to have fewer friends, and to find it more difficult to make friends. Hearing-impaired respondents were not, however, less likely to enjoy casual chat with friends, workmates, and neighbours (Table 4.19A). Perhaps casual chat is highly predictable and redundant in content, and is therefore easier for hearing-impaired people to sustain. The second part of the table (4.19B) describes the relationship between psychological disturbance and social life items. The only strong degree of association is that between loneliness and the SAD. Having fewer friends and difficulty in making friends do not appear to be associated with stress as measured by the SAD. It may be the case that people in upper middle-age (two thirds of the sample are over 50) expect to have fewer friends and to find it more difficult to make friends irrespective of hearing loss. The item on loneliness is the odd one out because it is not really a "social" item. In fact, the wording of the question makes it clear that loneliness should not be thought of as being related to friendship:

> "We all have different ideas about what being lonely is. It may have very little to do with the number of friends you have or the number of people you know. Would you describe yourself as a lonely person?"

For a rather different interpretation of data on social life, see Gilhome Herbst (1980).

TABLE 4.19

A. Comparison between the Hearing Impaired and the NOP Matched Control Group on Items Relating to Social Life

| Item | Hearing impaired | NOP | $p^a$ |
|---|---|---|---|
| Feeling lonely | 24% (49 out of 208) | 15% (61 out of 418) | <.01 |
| Having few or no friends | 40% (82 out of 208) | 25% (104 out of 418) | <.001 |
| Finding it difficult or very difficult to make friends | 40% (84 out of 211) | 15% (64 out of 418) | <.001 |
| Does not enjoy casual chat or passing the time of day with friends, workmates, neighbours, and so on | 26% (53 out of 205) | 20% (85 out of 418) | NS |

B. Relationship Between Psychological Disturbance and Social Life

| | Section of sample | | |
|---|---|---|---|
| Item | Normal | SAD cases | $p^a$ |
| Being a lonely person | 15% (25 out of 165) | 62% (24 out of 39) | .001 |
| Having few or no friends | 36% (60 out of 165) | 55% (21 out of 38) | .05 |
| Difficult or very difficult to make friends | 39% (64 out of 166) | 49% (19 out of 39) | NS |
| Does not enjoy casual chat or passing the time of day with friends, workmates, neighbours, and so on | 26% (43 out of 166) | 26% (10 out of 39) | NS |

$^a$NS, Not significant.

## C. Family Life

Hearing loss is not associated with marital breakdown. Indeed, the proportion of the hearing impaired who were separated or divorced was similar to that in the Quality of Life Survey, and was actually slightly lower than in the NOP matched control group. Given this, the next question concerned the effect of hearing loss on the *quality* of married life, a notoriously difficult area to investigate. Respondents were simply asked whether they tended to have rows concerning various aspects of married life (items adapted from Bradburn, 1969). As Table 4.20 shows, there was no difference between the hearing impaired and the NOP matched control group.

TABLE 4.20

Comparison between the Hearing Impaired and NOP Matched Control Group for Rows
Concerning Various Aspects of Married Life

| Area of married life | Hearing impaired | NOP matched group | $\chi^2$ $(p)^a$ |
|---|---|---|---|
| Deciding whether to see friends together | 24% (37 out of 157) | 16% (52 out of 320) | NS |
| Getting on with neighbours | 6% (10 out of 156) | 11% (35 out of 321) | NS |
| Being overtired | 35% (54 out of 156) | 33% (105 out of 322) | NS |
| Getting on with in-laws | 24% (36 out of 149) | 19% (52 out of 273) | NS |
| Disciplining children | 41% (42 out of 102) | 36% (74 out of 205) | NS |
| Spouse not listening | 37% (57 out of 156) | 35% (114 out of 322) | NS |
| Going out together | 17% (27 out of 156) | 17% (53 out of 321) | NS |
| One partner not showing enough affection | 27% (42 out of 156) | 19% (60 out of 322) | <.05 |
| Nothing in particular | 35% (55 out of 156) | 43% (138 out of 321) | NS |

[a]NS, Not significant.

Items on marriage and family life in which mention was made of hearing loss could not, of course, be controlled on the general population. As might be expected from the comparisons in Table 4.20, psychological disturbance was not related to having rows (Table 4.21). However, questions concerning the overall effect of hearing loss on marriage and family life were significantly associated with psychological disturbance, strongly suggesting that aspects of marriage and family life (not covered in this study) are very much affected by hearing loss.

TABLE 4.21

Relationship between the SAD and Items Concerning Marriage and Family Life[a]

| Items | Normal | SAD cases | $\chi^2$ $(p)^b$ |
|---|---|---|---|
| Having rows arising from deafness | 40% (52 out of 129) | 48% (12 out of 25) | NS |
| Deafness adversely affects marriage | 20% (26 out of 130) | 60% (15 out of 25) | <.001 |
| Deafness significantly affects family life | 30% (48 out of 158) | 54% (20 out of 37) | <.01 |

[a]These are items which could not be controlled on the general population.
[b]NS, Not significant.

## VII. CHARACTERISTICS OF THE "SEVERELY HEARING-IMPAIRED" SUBSAMPLE

It will be recalled that the 23 respondents in this subsample had hearing losses of 70 dB or greater, in conjunction with poor speech discrimination scores of 70% or less. The demographic structure of the group is given in Table 4.22. The age distribution does not differ greatly from the age distribution of the sample as a whole, in that 57% are over the age of 50, compared with 66% for the sample as a whole. The small imbalance is due mainly to more young females (under 40) than would be expected in the severely hearing-impaired subsample. If men over 60 years of age are excluded, the ratio of women to men is exactly 2:1, while for the sample as

TABLE 4.22

Demographic Structure of Severely Hearing Impaired Group[a]

*Age and sex distribution of the "severely hearing impaired" subsample*

| | | | Age | | |
|---|---|---|---|---|---|
| | 39 | 40–49 | 50–59 | 60–64 | Total |
| Male | 1 | 2 | 3 | 5 | 11 |
| Female | 5 | 2 | 5 | — | 12 |
| Total | 6 | 4 | 8 | 5 | 23 |

*Social class distribution*

| | I | II | IIIN | IIIM | IV | V |
|---|---|---|---|---|---|---|
| N | 2 | 4 | 5 | 5 | 3 | 2 |

*Mean dB loss*

| | 70–79 | 80–89 | 90–99 | 100+ |
|---|---|---|---|---|
| N | 10 | 3 | 5 | 5 |

*Type of loss*

| Sensorineural | "Mixed" | Conductive |
|---|---|---|
| 18 | 3 | 2 |

[a]The "severely hearing impaired" subsample has a mean loss of 70 dB or more, and a speech discrimination score of 70% or less.

TABLE 4.23

Distribution of the ''Severely Hearing Impaired'' Subsample amongst the
Three Hearing Aid Clinics that Constituted the Sample

| Hospital | Percentage of ''severely hearing impaired'' | Distribution of SAD cases |
|---|---|---|
| 1 (inner London) | 8% (6 out of 79) | 3 out of 5 |
| 2 (outer suburb) | 11% (10 out of 89) | 4 out of 9 |
| 3 (inner suburb) | 16% (7 out of 43) | 5 out of 7 |
| Overall | 11% (23 out of 211) | 12 out of 21 |

a whole, the distribution is roughly equal. That the subsample contains few
with conductive hearing losses is to be expected.

Table 4.23 gives the distributions of (a) the ''severe'' group across the
three hearing aid clinics, and (b) the distribution of SAD cases within each
group for each hearing aid clinic taken separately. There is no reason to
believe that the subsample was particularly located at any one hearing aid
clinic, either with regard to being a member of the subsample (based on
having a severe hearing impairment), or with regard to being a SAD case.

The ''severe'' group differed from the rest of the sample in the predicted
direction on almost all variables measured in the study. Out of the 42
psychological, social, and health variables, only five were not significantly
different in the predicted direction. In comparisons with the rest of the
sample, the subsample was *not:*

    More likely to be unemployed
    More likely to be left out of family decision-making
    More likely to suffer a further physical disability or health trouble
    More likely to have consulted a doctor concerning a nervous problem
    Less likely to have enough energy for day-to-day activities.

The other 37 measures all support the finding that the subsample is
indeed an extreme group. Table 4.24 gives 13 of the 37 discrete questions
that demonstrated especially large differences between the subsample and
the rest of the sample.

Finally, although the interview schedule consisted almost entirely of
closed questions, the interviewers from time to time did add spontaneous
comments of their own. The following is a selection of such comments

TABLE 4.24

Comparison of the "Severely Hearing Impaired" Subsample with the Rest of the Sample[a]

|  | Subsample (%) | Rest of sample (%) |
| --- | --- | --- |
| *Employment* |  |  |
| Changed job due to deafness | 24 | 10 |
| Hearing loss affects work a lot | 38 | 16 |
| Unhappy at work | 63 | 26 |
| *Social life* |  |  |
| No friends | 17 | 4 |
| Difficult to make friends | 18 | 5 |
| *Family life* |  |  |
| Separated/divorced | 13 | 2 |
| Deafness affects marriage | 53 | 24 |
| *Health* |  |  |
| Trouble in getting to sleep | 55 | 35 |
| Worry a great deal in general | 52 | 22 |
| Worry about a nervous breakdown | 24 | 6 |
| *As rated by interviewer* |  |  |
| Poor emotional state | 35 | 12 |
| Poor cooperation at interview | 13 | 2 |
| Hearing loss interfered severely with communication | 57 | 13 |

[a]These comparisons were made on items for which there is a large degree of difference. All the comparisons shown in this table are significant ($p < .01$).

made about those respondents who were eventually placed in the "severely hearing impaired" subsample.

"Had a feeling he did not understand and answer all the questions properly." (Man, 61, normal, i.e., aged 61 and identified as normal on the SAD)

"She believes you have to be really deaf before you realise what it's like to be deaf. Had to change her job from nursery nurse because she could not understand the children." (Woman, 51, SAD case, i.e., identified as disturbed)

"He was very aggressive and unpleasant at first, but gradually became chatty and sorry for himself; he was nearly in tears several times." (Man, 28, SAD case)

"The son-in-law brought this patient to the hospital—says he is *very* difficult to get on with." (Man, 57, SAD case)

"Extremely worried about his deafness and is desperate to have an operation to put everything right again. Seems to be pinning all his hopes on a miracle cure." (Man, 55, SAD case)

"She does not appear to realise the severity of her deafness . . . she does not hear and tries to compensate by guessing; it was difficult to assess whether she really understood some of the questions; sometimes she answered with some totally irrelevant remark." (Woman, 51, SAD case)

"Very little communication with anyone apart from her employer; an intelligent and very articulate person, very much in need of friends and companionship." (Woman, 28, SAD case)

"Deafness caused her to fail her clerical examination; has had to change her job for less responsibility and less money." (Woman, 28, SAD case)

"In past 7 years, has tried all sorts of ways of seeking help with his problem, from faith healing to acupuncture. Now accepts he is permanently deaf and has learned to control his anger and aggression, and channels his energy into learning, reading, and writing." (Man, 44, SAD case)

Many respondents in the subsample, however, were not psychologically disturbed. On the contrary, they appeared to have adjusted very well to hearing impairment:

"A man with few worries and few responsibilities." (Man, 44, normal)

"A good lip-reader; has worked as a "Samaritan," and still does!" (Man, 61, normal)

## VIII. THE NATURE OF HEARING HANDICAP

There is little doubt that hearing loss is associated with psychological disturbance, even though a number of years may have elapsed since the prescription of a hearing aid. On the other hand, no clear insights were obtained into the handicapping nature of hearing loss. In other words, the study served the actuarial purpose of quantifying psychological disturbance without throwing any light on what it was about living with hearing loss, which predisposed the sufferers to become psychologically disturbed. Hearing-impaired individuals were not more likely to be separated or divorced, nor were they more likely to be unemployed. Nevertheless, they were more worried about work, and unhappier at work. They also believed, generally speaking, that hearing loss had had an adverse effect on marriage and family life. As Table 4.25 shows, they perceived life in general to be less satisfying, in the past, present, and future. Unfortunately, the bulk of individual items related to family life and to work did not discriminate the hearing impaired from the control groups, and thus did not serve to show just how the quality of family, social, and working life was

TABLE 4.25

Comparison of Overall Life Satisfaction between the Hearing Impaired
Sample and Quality of Life Survey[a]

| Item | Significance level |
| --- | --- |
| Satisfaction with life five years ago | $p < .001$ |
| Satisfaction with life now | $p < .001$ |
| Expected satisfaction with life in five years' time | $p < .005$ |

[a]These comparisons were made using GLIM Analyses of Deviance, controlling for age and sex.

being affected. All that was learned was that hearing-impaired individuals had fewer friends and found it more difficult to make friends.

In order to examine the extent to which the hearing impaired themselves perceived acquired hearing loss to be a handicap, respondents were asked whether they considered themselves to be handicapped persons.

"People have different ideas about what makes somebody a handicapped person. Someone who is confined to a wheelchair is obviously handicapped, while someone who needs a walking stick may or may not be handicapped."

"A person who is completely blind is handicapped, while someone who is prevented from having a driving license because of poor eyesight may or may not be thought of as handicapped."

"Do you consider that having a hearing loss makes you yourself a handicapped person?"

From Table 4.26, it will be seen that the question divided the sample roughly into two halves, 98 respondents (43%) admitting to handicap. Perceiving oneself as handicapped by hearing loss was not related to being psychologically disturbed. The main purpose of this question, however, was to relate the item on handicap to other items, in order to learn more about the handicapping nature of acquired hearing loss. Surprisingly, the item was found to be unrelated to almost all others. Even its relationship with mean dB loss, while statistically significant, was minimal. Adjusted mean dB loss (controlling for age, sex, and social class) was 56 dB for those who admitted to handicap and 52 dB for those who did not. The same held for aided speech discrimination ability, controlling for dB loss, 76% phonemes correct for those who considered themselves handicapped, and 82% for those who did not. While these trends are consistent, they can

TABLE 4.26

Relationship between Feeling Handicapped by Hearing Loss and
Psychological Disturbance Measured by the SAD[a]

|  | Whether or not handicapped | |
| Result of SAD | Yes | No |
| --- | --- | --- |
| Normal section of sample | 77 | 88 |
| SAD cases | 21 | 18 |
| Total | 98 (43%) | 106 (57%) |
| % SAD cases | 21% | 17% |

[a] $\chi^2 < 1$; NS.

hardly be described as behaviourally significant. Virtually none of the psychological and psychosocial items were related to the handicap question, including those in which reference was made to hearing loss.

A possible interpretation as to why there is no relationship between psychological disturbance or other psychological/psychosocial variables and feeling handicapped by hearing loss is that many respondents may not have considered the possibility of a link between the two. They may have felt a deterioration in the quality of their lives without attributing it to hearing loss. They might have viewed increased feelings of anxiety, depression, and loneliness as consequences of other life experiences, such as ageing, for example. There is support for this interpretation in a study by Barcham and Stephens (1980), who found that very few people spontaneously mentioned emotional problems directly arising from hearing loss. Care should be taken, therefore, to ensure that hearing-impaired people are made aware of the very gradual and insidious effects that hearing loss may have on the quality of their lives.

Finally, any doubts as to whether hearing loss constitutes a significantly handicapping condition can be dispelled by comparison with a study which examined the incidence of psychological disturbance among the physically disabled (Garrad, 1975; Dongen Garrad, 1978). This study is especially interesting because an earlier version of the SAD was used (Foulds and Hope, 1968). Table 4.27 presents a comparison of the two studies. For those who are physically disabled, but for whom mobility is relatively unaffected, the proportion identified as psychologically disturbed is similar to that for the large majority of the hearing-impaired sample described in

TABLE 4.27

Comparative Effects of Physical Disability and Hearing Loss on Psychological Disturbance

Physical disability (using an earlier version of the SAD)

| | General population, based on normative data | Moderate restriction on mobility | Severe restriction on mobility |
| --- | --- | --- | --- |
| Proportion psychologically disturbed | 8% | 19% (16 out of 83) | 37% (43 out of 115) |

Hearing loss (based on SAD)

| | General population, based on normative data | Moderately hearing impaired | Severely hearing impaired |
| --- | --- | --- | --- |
| Proportion psychologically disturbed | 5% | 15% (27 out of 182) | 57% (12 out of 21) |

the table as moderately hearing impaired. Those with ''severe'' hearing loss (defined above) appear to be at least as likely to be psychologically disturbed as are the physically disabled, for whom mobility is severely restricted.

# PART THREE

*The Second Study:*
*Severe Sensorineural Hearing Loss*

# CHAPTER FIVE

## *Methodology and Audiological Characteristics*

### I. OBJECTIVES

The main objectives of the Second Study were as follows:

1. To test further the hypothesised link between severe hearing loss and psychological disturbance.
2. To investigate in greater depth the relationship between speech discrimination ability and psychological disturbance.
3. To test the hypothesis that the personality of hearing-impaired individuals does not differ from that of the normally hearing. (Evidence from personality studies of the physically disabled supports this hypothesis; moreover, the First Study showed that hearing-impaired respondents were not suspicious. The next step was to see whether there were *any* personality differences.)
4. To examine in greater depth the effect of hearing loss on employment.
5. To investigate the handicapping nature of hearing loss in greater detail, using the Hearing Measurement Scale (Noble and Atherley, 1970).
6. To explore the effect of hearing loss on family life, through home-based interviews with the families of hearing-impaired respondents.
7. To try out different approaches to the measurement of onset of hearing loss and to the quantification of hearing aid benefit.

### II. METHODOLOGY

#### A. Sample

All hearing aid clinics in the Greater London area were contacted, with the exception of those three that had participated in the First Study. Seven

103

were able to participate. A few did not participate for practical reasons, and one gave permission too late, after data collection had been completed. The target sample consisted of adults of employment age who had attended the hearing aid clinic for the first time between 1970 and 1978, and who had a sensorineural hearing loss of 60 dB or greater, averaged across the speech frequencies 0.5, 1, 2, and 4 kHz. After searching through records at these clinics, it soon became clear that the vast majority of the sample would be obtained from just one clinic, the Royal National Throat, Nose, and Ear Hospital, London.

A response rate of 51% resulted in a final sample of 88. See page 54 for a discussion of nonresponders.

## B.  Data Collection

All aspects of data collection were thoroughly piloted, firstly, on a group of severely hearing-impaired adults attending lipreading classes, and secondly, on respondents from the First Study who had a severe hearing loss. Each respondent was invited by letter to attend an interview at the hearing aid clinic from which he or she had originally obtained a hearing aid. Interviews were conducted by myself and by two research staff appointed to the project. The research staff was trained by a qualified audiometrician. The interview session lasted for around an hour and a half. Interviewing took place between August, 1979, and January, 1980. Collection of data followed the order given below.

### 1. *Audiometry*

Hearing loss in both ears was measured, air and bone, at 0.5, 1, 2, and 4 kHz. As type of hearing loss was not routinely included on the hearing aid clinic record card, it was necessary to measure bone conduction in order to exclude those cases with conductive or mixed hearing losses.

### 2. *Speech Discrimination*

a. *Boothroyd PB Word Lists.*    Details of this test are given on page 55. In the Second Study, two lists were administered, instead of one as in the

First Study. The test was administered under similar conditions, except that output was at 70 dB instead of 65 dB  as in the First Study. This slight concession to the marked difference in hearing loss between the two studies was made after a pilot study in which it was apparent that a large proportion would fail to score at all if the level were at 65 dB(A).

b. *SPIN Test.*    In order to investigate the relationship between speech discrimination and psychological variables in greater depth, an audiovisual version of the Speech Perception in Noise (SPIN) test was administered (Kalikow *et al.*, 1977). The main purpose of this test was to obtain a measure of speech discrimination ability under more natural conditions. As Hutcherson *et al.* (1979) put it:

> The purpose of the SPIN materials is to test speech reception using sentences that simulate a range of contextual situations encountered in everyday speech communication, [and] represents a significant departure from the typical clinical assessment of speech discrimination with monosyllabic words, where the emphasis is on the measurement of the acoustic–phonetic elements in speech [p. 239].

The SPIN test is made up of eight equivalent forms of 50 sentences each and is presented in noise (continuous babble). The task of the listener is to write down or repeat the key word which is the final word in each sentence (always a monosyllabic noun). The frequency of occurrence of key words is between 5 and 150 per million words, that is, in the middle range of the Thorndike Lorge word count (Thorndike and Lorge, 1944).

Twenty-five key words in each list have a high predictability (PH), and 25, a low predictability (PL). Thus, two scores emerge from the presentation of a list: a PH score and a PL score. A typical PH word is "fleet," as in "The admiral controls the fleet," and a typical PL word is "dent," as in "David has discussed the dent." The list chosen for this study was List 2.6. It was chosen as the one with the least Americanisms. Following trials with British subjects, only one item had to be altered, in which "cake" was substituted for "fudge," to read "I ate a piece of chocolate cake."

The audiovisual presentation was made with a Sony U-matic videotape recorder, and a 9-inch black and white monitor, with sound output from a single speaker placed directly below the monitor. Speech was set at 70 dB(A), and noise consisting of "cocktail babble" at 60 dB(A). The respondent was seated 1 m in front of the monitor.

Colour presentation was considered, but not used for a number of technical and practical reasons. McCormick (1980) has since shown that there is no difference in speechreading scores between colour and monochrome presentation. Incidentally, he has also shown that video presentation does not degrade lipreading scores in comparison with live presentation (Mc-Cormick, 1979b).

## 3. *Hearing Measurement Scale (HMS)*

The HMS (Noble and Atherley, 1970; Noble, 1971, 1978) is divided into seven sections representing different facets of handicap. From Table 5.1, it can be seen that scores from each section do not contribute equally to the overall score. The weightings are not psychometrically derived, however, but appear to reflect the judgement of the scale's authors. Nevertheless, it is the only scale of its kind which has been developed from interviews with "at risk" groups, ranging from bus drivers to boilermakers, and further refined following home interviews with people known to suffer sensorineural hearing losses. The scale was finally standardised on 27 hearing-impaired foundrymen (13 moulders, 8 grinders, and 6 chippers).

The HMS was administered in accordance with the author's instructions (Noble, 1972). Following pilot studies, a number of items were modified slightly to become acceptable for people with severe to profound hearing losses, leaving out words such as "ever," "never" and "always." For example:

Item 4: Do you (ever) have difficulty in group conversation outside?
Item 8: Can you (always) hear what's being said in a TV programme?

TABLE 5.1

Structure of the Hearing Measurement Scale (HMS)

| Section | Number of items | Maximum score |
|---|---|---|
| 1. Hearing for speech | 11 | 76 |
| 2. Hearing for nonspeech sound | 8 | 28 |
| 3. Spatial localisation | 7 | 28 |
| 4. Emotional response | 7 | 45 |
| 5. Speech distortion | 3 | 20 |
| 6. Tinnitus | 3 | 16 |
| 7. Personal opinion | 3 | 13 |
| Total | 42 | 226 |

For a similar reason, the word "hearing" was left out of the first two items in the scale:

> Item 1: Do you have difficulty in (hearing) conversation when you're with one other person when you're at home?
>
> Item 2: Do you have difficulty in (hearing) conversation when you're with one other person outside?

Finally, "car" was substituted for "motor," and "kettle" for "pan." The full, amended questionnaire is contained in Table 6.3

### 4. Self-completion Questionnaire

This is given in full in Appendix B. Briefly, it was concerned with the collection of demographic and biographical information, with data on cause and onset of hearing loss, and on hearing aid usage. A section covering problems encountered at work was also included; ideally such problems would have been explored in depth by interview, but this might have proved fatiguing, because respondents had already been exposed to a long interview (HMS), and various speech and hearing tests.

The last item of the Self-completion Questionnaire invited respondents to agree "in principle" to be interviewed at home with other members of their family present. This was the starting point for the Family Study, described in detail in Chapter 6.

### 5. Personality and Psychological Disturbance

Finally, respondents completed the Eysenck Personality Questionnaire (Eysenck and Eysenck, 1975) and the SAD, the measure of psychological disturbance (Scales of Anxiety and Depression) used in the First Study.

Interviewing took place between August, 1979, and January, 1980.

### III. CHARACTERISTICS OF THE SAMPLE

The final sample, following the exclusion of 37 respondents who were too old or prelingually deaf, or who had conductive or mixed losses, was comprised of 88 adults of employment age, with a mean dB loss of 60+ dB in the better ear, across the frequencies 0.5, 1, 2, and 4kHz. The majority of the sample, 69 out of 88, came from the Royal National Throat, Nose, and Ear Hospital. This was not caused by differential response rates, but simply reflected the fact that the hospital appeared to obtain the most referrals in the target category. The demographic structure of the sample is given in Table 5.2. There is a social class bias towards the upper social classes, similar to that found in the First Study.

There was, as expected, a marked age bias. There was no evidence of

TABLE 5.2

Demographic Structure of the Sample

*Hearing loss*

|  | Age | | | | |
|---|---|---|---|---|---|
|  | ≤39 | 40–49 | 50–59 | 60–64 | Total |
| Males | 3 | 9 | 22 | 17 | 51 |
| Females | 3 | 13 | 21 | — | 37 |
| Total | 6 | 22 | 43 | 17 | 88 |

*Social class*

|  | I and II | IIIN | IIIM | IV and V | Housewife |
|---|---|---|---|---|---|
| Males | 14 | 8 | 16 | 13 | — |
| Females | 7 | 13 | 3 | 8 | 6 |
| Total | 21 (24%) | 21 (24%) | 19 (21%) | 21 (24%) | 6 (7%) |

*Employment status*

|  | Males | Females | Total |
|---|---|---|---|
| Employment | 37 | 24 | 61 |
| Self-employed | 6 | 0 | 6 |
| Unemployed | 3 | 1 | 4 |
| Retired | 3 | 0 | 3 |
| Not employed | 1 | 11 | 12 |
| No response | 1 | 1 | 2 |
| Total | 51 | 37 | 88 |

*Marital status*

|  | Males | Females | Total |
|---|---|---|---|
| Married | 39 | 21 | 60 |
| Single | 5 | 3 | 8 |
| Widowed | 1 | 5 | 6 |
| Divorced/separated | 5 | 8 | 13 |
| No response | 1 | — | 1 |
| Total | 51 | 37 | 88 |

unemployment, even in this severely impaired group. The proportion separated or divorced was very high: 15%, compared with 3% in the First Study.

## A. Hearing Loss Variables

### 1. *Mean dB Loss*

Distribution of hearing loss scores is given in Table 5.3. Mean hearing loss was 76 dB, with men being significantly less impaired than women. It does not seem, therefore, that noise-induced hearing loss, which is more likely to affect males, is as significantly a factor as it might have been if the study had been conducted in an area of heavy industry.

Table 5.4 gives the mean dB loss at each frequency for each ear. Overall, it is clear that hearing level deteriorates markedly at the higher frequencies.

Table 5.5 shows that, in this relatively homogeneous sample, at least, hearing loss does not increase with age. The correlation between mean dB loss and age was $-0.1$, and the correlation between mean dB loss at 4 kHz and age was $-0.06$ (right ear) and $-0.08$ (left ear). These correlations are minimal, and similar to those found in the First Study. Once again, it seems that postlingually impaired adults of working age are a distinct group, different from the general population or from the elderly hearing impaired, for whom degree of hearing loss does increase with age (Gilhome Herbst and Humphrey, 1981). The overall difference in hearing

TABLE 5.3

Distribution of Mean dB Loss in the Better Ear

| | Mean dB loss | | | | | |
|---|---|---|---|---|---|---|
| | 60–69 | 70–79 | 80–89 | 90–99 | 100+ | Mean |
| Males | 25 | 12 | 7 | 3 | 4 | 74 ($\pm$ 15) |
| Females[a] | 10 | 10 | 10 | 2 | 5 | 80 ($\pm$ 14) |
| Total | 35 | 22 | 17 | 5 | 9 | ($\bar{X} = 76 \pm 15$) |

[a]Mean dB loss for women was significantly greater ($p < .06$).

TABLE 5.4

Mean dB Loss at Each Frequency for Each Ear

| Frequency (kHz) | Right ear (SD) | Left ear (SD) |
|---|---|---|
| 0.5 | 66 (29) | 68 (24) |
| 1 | 75 (20) | 79 (20) |
| 2 | 86 (20) | 89 (20) |
| 4 | 97 (20) | 97 (22) |

loss for males and females, described above, appears consistent for all age groups.

Table 5.6 shows that, as expected, and as demonstrated by numerous investigations (e.g., D'Souza et al., 1975; MacAdam et al., 1981), there is a relationship between social class and hearing loss although it is not marked.

## 2. Onset of Hearing Loss

An attempt to establish age of onset of hearing loss with any degree of reliability in the First Study was unsuccessful, the only concrete conclusion being that most respondents waited a considerable number of years after experiencing hearing loss before consulting a doctor. Moreover, there was little agreement between the time perceived to elapse from onset of hearing loss to consultation with a general practitioner and time elapsed from onset to acquisition of an aid (see page 69). A similar picture emerged in the Second Study, in which the mean number of years which had elapsed

TABLE 5.5

Relationship between Age and Hearing Loss

| | Mean dB loss | | |
|---|---|---|---|
| | All frequencies | | |
| Age | Males (N) | Females (N) | At 4 kHz |
| ≤39 | 72 (3) | 88 (3) | 98 |
| 40–49 | 76 (9) | 84 (13) | 96 |
| 50–59 | 71 (22) | 75 (21) | 88 |
| 60–64 | 76 (17) | — | 91 |

TABLE 5.6

Relationship between Social Class and Hearing Loss

| | Mean dB loss ($N$) | |
|---|---|---|
| Social class | First study | Second study |
| I | 51   (16) | 70   (6) |
| II | 52   (47) | 73   (15) |
| IIIN | 55   (34) | 71   (21) |
| IIIM | 54   (70) | 76   (19) |
| IV | 57   (31) | 84   (13) |
| V | 66   (11) | 79   (8) |
| | (NS) | ($p < .01$) |

between onset and medical consultation was 6.0 years, and between onset and acquisition of an aid, 14.9 years. A possible interpretation is that people consult their doctor when their hearing starts to deteriorate, but do not feel the need to acquire an aid until some considerable time later, when further deterioration has presumably made it difficult to cope without amplification. This interpretation is supported by the fact that onset of hearing loss is extremely gradual in the majority of cases. On the other hand, while it should follow that those who experience sudden onset would obtain an aid relatively quickly, this was not, in fact, the case. As Table 5.7 illustrates, while those who experienced sudden loss did not wait long before consulting a doctor, they still waited an inordinately long time before acquiring an aid. Finally, the standard deviations indicate a great deal of variability, implying an almost total absence of any pattern.

TABLE 5.7

Effect of Nature of Onset of Hearing Loss on the Length of Time Which Elapses before a General Practitioner Is Consulted and before a Hearing Aid Is Obtained

| Nature of onset | Years elapsed before consulting general practitioner (SD) | Years elapsed before acquiring a hearing aid (SD) |
|---|---|---|
| Sudden ($N = 11$) | 1.2 (3.0) | 15.1 (13.4) |
| Gradual ($N = 12$) | 3.2 (7.7) | 9.0 (11.9) |
| Very gradual ($N = 52$) | 7.7 (9.9) | 15.6 (11.4) |

## 3. *The Hearing Aid*

In the First Study, the measurement of hearing aid benefit on the scale "always, often, sometimes, rarely, never," was found not to be very useful, in that it was not related to any other variables. When degree of benfit was measured by the increase in speech discrimination ability between unaided and aided listening conditions, those with sensorineural losses were shown to obtain very little or no apparent benefit from wearing an aid. In the Second Study, different approaches to the measurement of hearing aid benefit were adopted. Table 5.8 shows two of these approaches. Firstly, everyday usage of the aid was broken down into use at work, at home, in the street, and when alone. Secondly, respondents were asked to estimate the number of hours spent per day wearing the aid. As might be expected from a sample comprised mainly of those with severe hearing losses, the great majority did appear to persevere with their aids. However, it is clear from Table 5.8 that in neither case is there a clear relationship between usage and degree of hearing loss. While the sample is

TABLE 5.8

Use Made of Hearing Aid

| Amount of time worn in different situations[a] | At work | At home | In street | When alone |
|---|---|---|---|---|
| Never | 15 (71) | 11 (71) | 29 (74) | 24 (73) |
| Sometimes | 10 (71) | 24 (73) | 11 (75) | 12 (71) |
| Most of the time | 48 (77) | 53 (79) | 48 (78) | 49 (78) |
| Not applicable | 15 | — | — | 3 |

| Hours worn per day | $N$ | Hearing loss (dB)[b] |
|---|---|---|
| 0 | 12 | 71 |
| 1–4 | 7 | 78 |
| 5–8 | 9 | 72 |
| 9–12 | 13 | 87 |
| 13–16 | 37 | 77 |
| 17+ | 6 | 71 |
| Total | 84 | |

[a]dB loss in brackets; $N = 84$.
[b]Mean = 77 dB.

TABLE 5.9

Use Made of Hearing Aid Controlling for Other Variables

A. Analysis of Variance of the Number of Hours per Day during Which
the Hearing Aid is Worn[a]

| Source | df | SS | F | p |
|---|---|---|---|---|
| Sex | 1 | 130 | 3.4 | 0.07 |
| dB loss | 5 | 369 | 2.0 | 0.10 |
| Communication ability | 4 | 186 | 1.2 | NS |
| Age (covariate) | 1 | 1 | 0.02 | NS |
| Residual | 66 | 2484 | — | — |
| Total | 77 | 3116 | — | — |

B. Effect of Sex, dB Loss, and Communication Ability on Number of
Hours an Aid is Worn Daily[b]

| Main effect | Hours per day aid worn |
|---|---|
| Males | 9.4 |
| Females | 12.2 |
| Hearing loss (dB) | |
| 60–79 | 9.3 |
| 80–99 | 11.9 |
| 100–120 | 14.3 |
| Communication ability | |
| Poor | 8.0 |
| Neither poor nor good | 9.5 |
| Good | 11.9 |

[a] $N = 78$.
[b] Adjusted for other main affects and covariate of age.

to some extent homogeneous with reference to dB loss, it is nevertheless obvious that usage is largely determined by factors other than hearing ability for pure tones.

An Analysis of Variance of the number of hours per day during which the aid was worn was carried out in order to quantify the effect of sex, dB loss, and communication ability (Table 5.9). Communication ability was rated on a five-point scale by the interviewer at the end of the interview. As can be seen in part A of Table 5.9, the effects due to sex and dB loss have a borderline significance. The covariate of age was insignificant. Adjusted scores for the main effects are given in part B of this table. While communication ability does not have a significant effect on the number of hours, the trend is consistent with what would be expected. Those with profound hearing losses make greater use of the aid, which is surprising, given that people with profound losses are generally believed to obtain little or no benefit from hearing aid usage. On the other hand, the correlation between mean dB loss and hours per day the aid was worn ($r = .09$) was insignificant, indicating a massive variation in use made of the aid for all levels of hearing loss. Greater use of the hearing aid by men may be due to more use made of the hearing aid at work. In a separate Analysis of Variance, social class was not found to influence the number of hours the aid was worn.

### 4. Speech Discrimination

Two measures of speech discrimination ability were used. Boothroyd's PB Word Lists were used again, in order to see if a relationship between discrimination of speech and psychological disturbance held for a larger and more homogeneous sample. The SPIN Test was also administered, audiovisually, in order to obtain a measure of speech discrimination ability when visual and contextual clues were available. Frequencydistributions, means, and standard deviations are given in Table 5.10.

### 5. Relationship between Social Class and Speech Discrimination

Table 5.11 describes the surprising relationship between speech discrimination ability and social class, noted by Thomas and Ring (1984). The Boothroyd Word List scores are interdependent, because word and phoneme scores are derived from the same word lists.

Table 5.12 gives Analyses of Variance of the speech discrimination test scores by social class, along with tests for linear trend. Both the Boothroyd Tests and the SPIN Test (high probability condition) demonstrate a highly significant social class effect, though the SPIN Test (low probability condition) does not. However, all tests reveal a highly significant trend of linearity.

Every attempt was made to account for the relationship in terms of other factors. Mean dB loss obviously had a strong influence on speech scores,

TABLE 5.10

Frequency Distribution, Means, and Standard Deviations for Speech Discrimination Tests

A. *Boothroyd PB Word Lists*[a]

| % Words correct | N | Cumulative % |
|---|---|---|
| 0 | 22 | 27 |
| 1–20 | 22 | 54 |
| 21–40 | 25 | 84 |
| 41–60 | 1 | 95 |
| 61–80 | 4 | 100 |
| 81–100 | 0 | |

Mean words correct: 21.7 (SD = 20.2)

| % Phonemes correct | N | Cumulative % |
|---|---|---|
| 0 | 15 | 18 |
| 1–20 | 9 | 29 |
| 21–40 | 16 | 49 |
| 41–60 | 27 | 82 |
| 61–80 | 13 | 98 |
| 81–100 | 2 | 100 |

Mean words correct: 37.1 (SD = 25.0)

B. *SPIN Test*

| % Low probability words correct | N | Cumulative % |
|---|---|---|
| 0 | 16 | 20 |
| 1–20 | 12 | 35 |
| 21–40 | 30 | 72 |
| 41–60 | 20 | 96 |
| 61–80 | 3 | 100 |

Mean = 28.0 (SD = 20.0)

| % High probability words correct | N | Cumulative % |
|---|---|---|
| 0 | 11 | 14 |
| 1–20 | 5 | 20 |
| 21–40 | 3 | 23 |
| 41–60 | 15 | 42 |
| 61–80 | 21 | 68 |
| 81–100 | 19 | 100 |

Mean = 60.0 (SD = 32.0)

[a]Based on two lists.

TABLE 5.11

Effect of Social Class on Speech Discrimination Scores

| | Boothroyd monosyllabic word lists | | SPIN test | |
| Social class | Words mean (SD) | Phonemes mean (SD) | High probability words mean (SD) | Low probability words mean (SD) |
|---|---|---|---|---|
| I | 41.0 | 62.0 | 71.2 | 40.0 |
| II | 35.3 | 55.7 | 78.1 | 33.3 |
| IIIN | 24.7 | 41.5 | 66.3 | 31.4 |
| IIIM | 18.6 | 33.9 | 64.0 | 27.6 |
| IV | 11.5 | 20.5 | 38.5 | 20.0 |
| V | 8.3 | 20.2 | 31.2 | 19.2 |
| Overall means: | 22.9 (20.2) | 38.5 (25.0) | 61.3 (31.6) | 28.6 (19.7) |

but did not affect the relationship between speech and social class. Other variables affecting speech scores but not the relationship between speech and social class were (a) wearing the hearing aid for the speech test, (b) wearing a hearing aid at work, and (c) psychological disturbance. In the light of Bergman's work (Bergman et al., 1976), it is rather surprising that age did not influence speech scores, though this may have been due to the homogeneity of the sample with regard to age. Davis (1983) has reported a similar finding, though without offering any explanation for it.

In the light of the above, we decided to reanalyse the speech and social class data obtained during the course of the First Study, in which a straightforward Analysis of Variance of speech scores had revealed no effect due to social class. As Table 5.13 shows, there is a discernible trend, though by no means as marked as those in the Second Study. The Analysis of Variance in Table 5.14 confirms that the relationship is much weaker, though the test for linearity in the aided condition is highly significant.

Overall, there is little doubt that speech discrimination scores are influenced by social class independently of other factors known to influence speech discrimination. Moreover, the consistency of the trend from group to group is remarkable. The obvious explanation which comes to mind centres on class differences in linguistic ability (Bernstein, 1971; Fillmore

TABLE 5.12

One-way Analyses of Variance of Speech Discrimination Scores by Social Class with Tests for Linear Trends

| A. *Boothroyd Word Score* | | | | |
| Source | *SS* | *df* | *MS* | *p* |
| --- | --- | --- | --- | --- |
| Between | 7,310 | 5 | 1,462 | 0.002 |
| Within | 23,812 | 71 | 335 | — |
| Test for linearity | | | | 0.001 |
| Tests for nonlinearity | | | | NS |
| B. *Boothroyd Phoneme Score* | | | | |
| Source | *SS* | *df* | *MS* | *p* |
| Between | 14,004 | 5 | 2,801 | 0.001 |
| Within | 33,620 | 71 | 474 | — |
| Test for linearity | | | | 0.001 |
| Tests for nonlinearity | | | | NS |
| C. *SPIN Test (High Probability)* | | | | |
| Source | *SS* | *df* | *MS* | *p* |
| Between | 16,668 | 5 | 3,334 | 0.003 |
| Within | 58,417 | 70 | 835 | — |
| Test for linearity | | | | 0.001 |
| Tests for nonlinearity | | | | NS |
| D. *SPIN Test (Low Probability)* | | | | |
| Source | *SS* | *df* | *MS* | *p* |
| Between | 2,560 | 5 | 512 | NS |
| Within | 26,529 | 70 | 379 | — |
| Test for linearity | | | | 0.02 |
| Tests for nonlinearity | | | | NS |

*et al.*, 1979). However, none of the linguistic abilities described by these writers would serve to explain differences in the ability to hear very simple, monosyllabic, everyday words at or near the threshold of hearing, especially when there are no contextual clues which would favour those more highly developed linguistic abilities. It is also unlikely that the method of scoring has anything to do with the effect. In the First Study, the respondent called out the responses and the interviewer wrote them down, and in the Second Study, the respondent wrote them down. The effect,

TABLE 5.13

Effect of Social Class on Speech Discrimination Ability Based on Data
from the First Study

| Social class | Boothroyd monosyllabic word list | |
|---|---|---|
| | Unaided means | Aided means |
| I | 61.4 | 80.3 |
| II | 65.1 | 82.8 |
| IIIN | 58.6 | 78.1 |
| IIIM | 52.3 | 79.0 |
| IV | 50.1 | 77.5 |
| V | 35.7 | 62.6 |
| Overall mean | 56.2 (SD = 33.2) | 78.0 (SD = 26.5) |

therefore, appears to hold for the two methods of scoring. An instruction
common to both studies was to exhort the respondent to "have a stab" at
the word, however unsure he or she was about it, and to repeat or write
down any part of the word which had been heard. It is thus possible that
there are class differences related to willingness to "have a stab," rather
than to ability to discriminate speech. This should be relatively easy to

TABLE 5.14

One-way Analyses of Variance of Speech Discrimination Scores by Social Class with
Tests for Linear Trends, Based on Data from the First Study

| A. *Boothroyd Phoneme Score (Unaided)* Source | SS | df | MS | p |
|---|---|---|---|---|
| Between | 11,087 | 5 | 2,217 | 0.1 |
| Within | 234,818 | 201 | 1,169 | — |
| Test for linearity | | | | 0.005 |
| Tests for nonlinearity | | | | NS |
| B. *Boothroyd Phoneme Score (Aided)* Source | SS | df | MS | p |
| Between | 3,370 | 5 | 674 | NS |
| Within | 111,489 | 181 | 616 | — |
| Test for linearity | | | | 0.1 |
| Tests for nonlinearity | | | | NS |

control in a signal detection-type experiment utilising both verbal and nonverbal stimuli.

The validity of speech tests can obviously be improved if scores are weighted to accomodate the influence of social class. Such a procedure might be useful for research purposes, but has little value in individual cases, when an assessment is being made for the prescription of a hearing aid or for a rehabilitation programme (cf. the large standard deviations found for all the speech tests). What is more important, I believe, is that this finding gives further weight to Noble's contention (Noble, 1978) that speech tests do not reflect performance in real-life situations and that subjective estimates of speech performance are far more likely to be valid, simply because they will be based on real-life experience. Research needs to be carried out to compare speech test performance and subjective estimation of speech discrimination ability with performance in real-life situations. It would also be interesting to know if the relationship between speech discrimination and social class applies to normally hearing people when speech is presented around threshold.

# CHAPTER SIX

*Psychological and Psychosocial Effects*

## I. EFFECT OF SEVERE SENSORINEURAL
## HEARING LOSS ON PERSONALITY

The Eysenck Personality Questionnaire (EPQ) was administered to test the hypothesis that severe hearing loss does not cause any change in basic personality structure (Thomas, 1981a). This hypothesis directly contradicts earlier work reviewed in detail in Chapter 2. To recapitulate, Welles (1932) noted that those who appeared unable to adjust successfully to hearing loss were significantly more emotional, introverted, and less dominant than a hearing control group, based on the Bernreuter Personality Inventory. Nett (1960) and Myklebust (1964) found evidence of personality change on almost all of the MMPI scales, and Cattell *et al.* (1970) found a similar departure from normal on a number of the 16 PF scales. Stephens (1980) reported significantly elevated scores for introversion and neuroticism on the Eysenck Personality Inventory. These studies, however, shared a number of weaknesses, discussed in detail in Chapter 2. Their findings are also at variance with studies which have examined the effect of physical disability on personality (Shontz, 1970). Another reason behind the decision to administer a personality test derived from the conclusion, reached in Chapter 2, that there was no substantial evidence in support of the supposed association between hearing loss and paranoid mental states. If, however, there is any substance to the claim that hearing loss is associ-

TABLE 6.1

Comparison of the Hearing-Impaired Group with General Population Norms
on the Eysenck Personality Questionnaire

A. *Overall*

| Scale | General population means[a] (SD) | Means for the hearing impaired group[b] (SD) | p |
|---|---|---|---|
| Extraversion | 11.43 (5.06) | 10.30 (4.68) | NS |
| Neuroticism | 10.76 (5.38) | 11.49 (5.51) | NS |
| Psychoticism | 2.50 (2.32) | 2.56 (2.07) | NS |
| Lie Scale | 9.80 (4.42) | 10.91 (4.99) | NS |

B. *Broken down by age and sex*

| Scale | General population means[c] (SD) | Means for the hearing impaired group[d] (SD) | p |
|---|---|---|---|
| Extraversion | | | |
| male | 11.08 (5.14) | 11.40 (4.53) | NS |
| female | 11.86 (4.96) | 8.97 (4.57) | .01 |
| Neuroticism | | | |
| male | 9.45 (5.39) | 10.17 (5.30) | NS |
| female | 12.33 (5.36) | 13.09 (5.41) | NS |
| Psychoticism | | | |
| male | 2.70 (2.53) | 3.05 (2.16) | NS |
| female | 2.27 (2.03) | 1.97 (1.82) | NS |
| Lie scale | | | |
| male | 9.52 (4.43) | 9.62 (4.83) | NS |
| female | 10.13 (4.40) | 12.46 (4.80) | .03 |

[a]General population norms are adjusted to match the age and sex structure
of the hearing-impaired sample.

[b]$N = 77$.

[c]General population norms are adjusted to match the age structure of the
hearing-impaired sample.

[d]42 males and 35 females.

ated with paranoid mental states, then EPQ scores on the dimensions of
neuroticism and psychoticism would be expected to be markedly elevated.

Means for the three personality dimensions of the EPQ and for the Lie
Scale are given in part A of Table 6.1. The general population norms in the

table are derived from the ones published in the EPQ manual, adjusted to match the age and sex structure of the hearing-impaired sample. The hearing-impaired group did not differ significantly from general population norms on any of the four EPQ scales. The differences between means for the Extraversion and Lie Scales, while not statistically significant, were large enough ($p < .1$) to merit further examination. Comparisons between the hearing-impaired group with norms for each of the personality variables and for the Lie Scale were then broken down by sex (Table 6.1, part B). It emerged that hearing-impaired females were significantly more introverted and also had significantly elevated Lie Scale scores.

The authors of the EPQ point out that the Lie Scale is indicative of dissimulation only when there is a relatively high correlation with neuroticism, "which approaches, or is greater than 0.5." In this study, the overall correlation between the two scales was $-0.19$, which while statistically significant, is very low, accounting for less than 4% of the variance. The correlation for females taken separately was $-0.18$. The elevated Lie Scale score for females can therefore be discounted with regard to any possible influence on the personality dimensions.

These findings, which are at variance with earlier studies mentioned above, support the hypothesis that basic personality structure is relatively unaffected, even by severe hearing loss. They are, however, in accord with findings from studies of the effect of physical disability on personality, reviewed by Shontz (1970).

The sample for this study was drawn from the extreme end of the hearing-impairment spectrum. Hearing loss was sensorineural, and ranged from moderately severe to total. (Severity of loss was not a significant factor.) Moreover, all respondents were of employment age and thus likely to experience the maximum adverse effect of hearing loss at work and at home. Such factors could serve as the basis for believing that personality deviations would be more marked than in the other studies which were, almost without exception, based on less-impaired individuals. Nevertheless, basic personality structure was not affected by hearing loss. The only comparison contained in Table 6.1 that shows a personality difference is for females who are significantly introverted. The very nature of extraversion should, more than any other personality variable, predispose the hearing impaired to obtain low scores. It would seem fair to conclude that the females in the sample are genuinely introverted, rather than that there is any misclassification due to the effects of hearing loss. It is surprising, therefore, that hearing-impaired males are not "introverted." The important scales, however, are those of neuroticism and psychoticism, for had there been any underlying personality disturbance or predisposition to a paranoid reaction, then the scores on these scales should have been markedly elevated, as the authors of the EPQ have pointed out (Eysenck and Eysenck, 1975).

In Chapter 2, the supposed association between hearing loss and paranoid mental states was shown to be unsubstantiated. Then, in the First Study, a measure of mild suspiciousness failed to discriminate hearing-impaired respondents from the general population. It now seems fair to conclude that hearing loss does not result in any longstanding personality change whatsoever. Incidentally, a recent community study based on an elderly population also found that personality disorder was unrelated to hearing loss (Gilhome Herbst and Humphrey, 1980).

## II. PSYCHOLOGICAL DISTURBANCE

Respondents in the First Study who had a severe hearing loss *and* poor speech discrimination scores were shown, as a group, to suffer a very high likelihood of psychological disturbance (see page 84). In the present study, out of a total sample of 88, 78 completed the psychological disturbance inventory, the SAD, and 14 (18%) were identified as disturbed. This compares with 12 out of 21 (57%) for those in the First Study who had a severe hearing loss as defined on page 93. (In the First Study as a whole, 19% were psychologically disturbed.) The only possible explanation appears in terms of systematic sample differences. It is unlikely that the finding in the First Study is a chance result—the trend was observed before interviewing at the first hearing aid clinic was completed, and manifested itself at both the second and the third hearing aid clinics taken separately (see page 94). One possible explanation is that the sample for the present study was concentrated in just one hospital that for some reason has treated a disproportionately high number of patients with severe sensorineural hearing loss.

It is not possible to explain the difference in the proportions of the

TABLE 6.2

The Relationship between Speech Discrimination and Psychological Disturbance

A. *Analysis of Variance of Speech Discrimination Scores[a]*

| Source | SS | df | f | p |
|---|---|---|---|---|
| Mean dB loss (covariate) | 16,754 | 1 | 43.6 | .001 |
| Psychological disturbance (main effect) | 2,139 | 1 | 5.6 | .02 |
| Residual | 26,925 | 70 | — | — |
| Total | 45,818 | 72 | — | — |

B. *Means for Hearing Loss and Speech Discrimination by Psychological Disturbance*

| Psychological disturbance | N | Hearing loss (dB) | Unadjusted phoneme scores (%) | Adjusted phoneme scores[b] (%) |
|---|---|---|---|---|
| No | 59 | 77 | 40 | 40 |
| Yes | 14 | 74 | 29 | 26 |

[a] % phonemes on Boothroyd Word Lists.
[b] Adjusted for the covariate of hearing loss.

psychologically disturbed in terms of speech discrimination ability. In the First Study, the poor speech discriminators scored less than 70% phonemes correct on the Boothroyd Word Lists, while in the Second Study *everyone* scored less than 70% correct, which would have led to an expectation of a markedly elevated incidence of psychological disturbance. On the other hand, speech discrimination ability was still significantly related to psychological disturbance, even though the pattern was different from that obtained in the First Study. Table 6.2, part A, contains an Analysis of Covariance of speech discrimination scores on the Boothroyd Word Lists. The covariate of mean dB loss obviously has a large effect on speech discrimination scores. After controlling for mean dB loss, there is still a significant relationship between speech discrimination ability and psychological disturbance as measured by the SAD. Social class, which was known to affect speech discrimination scores, was independent of psychological disturbance. Table 6.2, part B, gives the mean speech discrimination scores for the psychologically normal and psychologically disturbed sections of the sample. As might be expected from the small difference in dB loss, phoneme scores adjusted to take the covariate of mean dB loss into account hardly differ from the unadjusted scores. It seems, therefore, that the significant relationship between discrimination of monosyllabic words and psychological disturbance is confirmed. Parallel Analyses of Covariance, in which other variables were introduced, did not suppress the relationship. On the other hand, no relationship was found between the SAD and the SPIN Test in either the high or low probability conditions. Why the effect occurs only with words presented singly defies interpretation. That it holds across two independent studies means that it is probably valid. The relationship between speech discrimination ability and psychological disturbance clearly merits further investigation. It might be worth examining the effect of psychological disturbance on speech discrimination ability (speech presented around threshold) for normally hearing adults, to investigate the possibility that psychological disturbance is the independent, rather than the dependent, variable.

Apart from speech discrimination ability, as measured by Boothroyd Word Lists, psychological disturbance was related to very few other variables. It was not related to age, sex, or social class, mean dB loss, or in general, to hearing loss variables, including the HMS. An unusual finding concerned the 12 respondents who had suffered sudden onset of hearing loss, not one of whom was psychologically disturbed, giving some support to the suggestion that though more traumatic in the first instance, sudden onset of disability leads to better eventual adjustment than when it is gradual or very gradual Another unusual finding concerned the tinnitus section of the Hearing Measurement Scale, which, for some reason, was related to speech discrimination ability, though independently of psychological disturbance and social class. It seems, therefore, that tinnitus, psychological disturbance, and social class, as well as mean dB loss, all affect speech discrimination ability. Factors affecting speech discrimination ability clearly need further investigation.

Although severe hearing loss was not associated with a very high level of psychological disturbance, as in the First Study, hearing-impaired adults were still nearly four times more likely to be psychologically disturbed than were normally hearing people. This proportion was similar to that found in the First Study, although the two samples differed, especially with regard to severity of hearing loss. The picture is further complicated because while the proportion of psychological disturbance is not as high as expected, other variables indicative of stress show a markedly increased effect in the Second Study. In the First Study, seven out of 211 respondents (3.3%) were separated or divorced, a proportion similar to that found in the general population. In the Second Study, however, 13 out of 88 (14.7%) were separated or divorced. Moreover, of the 55 respondents in the Second Study who were working, 34 (62%) had suffered a loss of job status, whereas in the First Study, respondents did not feel that hearing loss had affected their promotion prospects or that their jobs were not commensurate with their abilities.

Finally, 50 (56%) respondents reported tinnitus, and 19 (22%) found it sometimes or always upsetting. However, as mentioned above, the condition was not associated with psychological disturbance, indicating that most sufferers are able to cope with it, and do not allow it to get them down unduly.

## III. SUBJECTIVE QUANTIFICATION OF HEARING HANDICAP (HMS)

While the HMS is the best-developed of the hearing handicap scales, it has been little-used, and not once with a sample of adults with severe sensorineural hearing loss. An item analysis was therefore undertaken in order to see whether the sections of the scale corresponded to separate areas of handicap (Table 6.3). The technique used was a factor analysis based on the first six sections of the HMS. Section Seven was omitted because one of the items was deemed unsuitable for a sample known to suffer severe hearing loss (item 40: "Do you think your hearing is normal?"). The intention was to produce the six factors which best accounted for the relationship between the items. Noble and Atherley (1970) have shown that, as might be predicted, the sections of the HMS are interrelated. Therefore, an oblique factor rotation was adopted. Where an item loads less than 0.3 ($p < .05$) on a factor, it is omitted (i.e., where the contribution of an item is insignificant). As Table 6.3 shows, in general, it was found that the factors which emerged corresponded to the first six sections of the HMS (Table 6.3). If we take HMS Section Three as an example, we see that items 20 to 23, and 25, all load on Factor III and on no other factor, indicating that HMS Section Three is well differentiated. Item 26, however, appears to be more related to HMS Section Two, although it does have a second highest loading on Factor III. Item 24,

TABLE 6.3

Relationship of Items to Factors Based on the First Six Sections of the HMS[a,b,c]

| Item | Factors | Loadings |
| --- | --- | --- |
| *Section One: Speech Hearing* | | |
| 1. Do you have difficulty in conversation when you're with one other person at home? | I | .40 |
| 2. Do you have difficulty in conversation when you're with one other person outside? | II | .50 |
| 3. Do you have difficulty in group conversation at home? | III | .40 |
| | (II) | (.36) |
| 4. Do you have difficulty in group conversation outside? | II | .46 |
| 5. Do you have difficulty hearing conversation normally demanded of you at work (or when travelling/shopping)? | I | .59 |
| 6. Do you have difficulty hearing the speaker at a public meeting? | — | — |
| 7. Can you hear what's being said in a TV programme? | I | .68 |
| | (V) | (.34) |
| 8. Can you hear what's being said in TV news? | I | .69 |
| 9. Can you head what's being said in a radio programme? | I | .84 |
| 10. Can you hear what's being said in radio news? | I | .86 |
| 11. Do you have difficulty hearing what's said in a film at the cinema? | I | .48 |
| *Section Two: Acuity for Nonspeech Sound* | | |
| 12. Do you have any pets at home? (Type _____) Can you hear it when it barks, mews, etc.? | — | — |
| 13. Can you hear when someone rings the doorbell or knocks on the door? | II | .37 |
| | (V) | (.34) |
| 14. Can you hear a car horn in the street when you're outside? | — | — |
| 15. Can you hear the sound of footsteps outside when you're inside? | II | .47 |
| 16. Can you hear the sound of the door opening when you're inside that room? | II | .65 |
| 17. Can you hear the clock ticking in the room? | II | .47 |
| 18. Can you hear the tap running when you turn it on? | II | .58 |
| 19. Can you hear water boiling in a kettle when you're in the kitchen? | II | .50 |
| *Section Three: Localisation* | | |
| 20. When you hear the sound of people talking and they're in another room, can you tell whereabouts this sound was coming from? | III | .65 |

(*continued*)

TABLE 6.3 (*Continued*)

| Item | Factors | Loadings |
|------|---------|----------|
| 21. If you're with a group of people and someone you can't see starts to speak, would you be able to tell where the person was sitting? | III | .72 |
| 22. If you hear a car horn or a bell can you always tell which direction it's sounding? | III | .52 |
| 23. Do you ever turn your head the wrong way when someone calls to you? | III | .64 |
| 24. Can you actually tell, from the sound, how far away a person is when he calls to you? | III (V) | .38 (.31) |
| 25. Have you ever noticed outside that a car you thought, by its sound, was far away turned out to be much closer? | III | .49 |
| 26. Outside, do you always move out of the way of something coming up from behind; for instance, a car, a trolley, or someone walking faster? | II (III) | .48 (.32) |
| *Section Four: Emotional Response* | | |
| 27. Do you think you are more irritable than other people, or less so? | IV | .53 |
| 28. Do you give the wrong answer to someone because you've misheard them? | II | .42 |
| 29. When you do this, do you treat it lightly or do you get upset? | IV | .76 |
| 30. How does the other person react? Does he get irritated or make little of it? | IV | .51 |
| 31. Do you think people are tolerant of your hearing difficulty, or do they make fun of you? | VI | .44 |
| 32. Do you ever get bothered or upset if you are unable to follow a conversation? | IV | .61 |
| 33. Do you ever get the feeling of being cutoff from things because of difficulty in hearing? | IV | .39 |
| *Section Five: Speech Distortion* | | |
| 34. Do you find that people fail to speak clearly? | V | .62 |
| 35. What about speakers on TV? Do they fail to speak clearly? | V | .57 |
| 36. Do you ever have difficulty in everyday conversation, understanding what someone is saying even though you can hear something is being said? | V | .40 |
| *Section Six: Tinnitus* | | |
| 37. Do you ever get a noise in your ears or in your head? | VI | .34 |
| 38. Does it ever keep you from sleeping? | VI | .52 |
| 39. Does it upset you? | VI | .69 |

[a]Table includes loadings of 0.3 or greater; $p < .05$.

[b]Second highest loadings on other factors, where appropriate, are given in parentheses.

[c]The HMS is reproduced by permission from Noble and Atherly (1970).

besides loading on Factor III, also loads on another factor. Evidence for the soundness of the HMS derives from the fact that (*a*) only five out of 39 items load significantly on more than one factor, (*b*) only three items do not load on any factor, and (*c*) only five items have loadings on factors which represent other HMS sections, three of which are in HMS Section One.

As stated, the items in HMS Section Seven were excluded from the main analysis because of the inappropriateness of item 40. A preliminary analysis, which included the remaining two items of HMS Section Seven (items 41 and 42), indicated that the section might not be well differentiated, because both items loaded significantly on other factors. Item 41 ("Do you think your hearing loss is a particularly serious one?") had a loading of .35 on Factor V; item 42 ("Does any difficulty with your hearing loss ever restrict your social and personal life?") had significant loadings on Factor V (.53) *and* Factor VI (.42).

TABLE 6.4

Correlations among HMS Factors and between HMS Sections and Factors

A. *Correlations among HMS Factors*

| Factors | I | II | III | IV | V |
|---|---|---|---|---|---|
| II | .40[a] | — | — | — | — |
| III | .34[a] | .38[a] | — | — | — |
| IV | .28[a] | .23 | .25[a] | — | — |
| V | .04 | .09 | .07 | .10 | — |
| VI | .15 | .14 | .04 | .01 | .05 |

B. *Correlations between HMS Sections and Factors*

HMS sections

| Factors | One | Two | Three | Four | Five | Six |
|---|---|---|---|---|---|---|
| I | .86[a] | .36[a] | .24 | .18 | .22 | .32[a] |
| II | .64[a] | .81[a] | .38[a] | .25[a] | .12 | .29[a] |
| III | .47[a] | .37[a] | .83[a] | .05 | .01 | .34[a] |
| IV | .31[a] | .10 | .19 | .68[a] | .11 | .16 |
| V | .26[a] | .08 | .01 | .24 | .79[a] | .06 |
| VI | .18 | .10 | .02 | .26 | .16 | .66[a] |

[a] $p < .05$.

TABLE 6.5

Comparison of HMS Mean Scores between Different Studies

| | Sections | | | | | | | |
|---|---|---|---|---|---|---|---|---|
| | One | Two | Three | Four | Five | Six | Seven | Total |
| Noble (1969) | 13 | 2 | 5 | 8 | 3 | 1 | 2 | 34 (*N* = 73) |
| Noble (1969) | 36 | 9 | 7 | 16 | 5 | 2 | 5 | 80 (*N* = 23) |
| Noble (1979) | 24 | 4 | 2 | 11 | 3 | 2 | 6 | 52 (*N* = 23, adapted from two subsamples of 11 and 12) |
| McCartney *et al.* (1976) | 29 | 6 | 9 | 13 | 6 | 1 | 5 | 69 (*N* = 36) |
| Stephens (1980) | 38 | 11 | 17 | 21 | 7 | 3 | 8 | 105 (*N* = 54) |
| Present study (pilot) | 45 | 15 | 18 | 14 | 6 | 4 | 8 | 110 (*N* = 13) |
| Present study | 39 | 12 | 15 | 19 | 7 | 2 | 11 | 105 (*N* = 88) |

Correlation within factors, and between factors and HMS sections, are given in Table 6.4. Overall, Factors I to IV are related, and Factors V and VI are independent. As expected, the correlations between factors and corresponding HMS sections is high. The overlap between the first four HMS sections and corresponding factors is also high. For a more detailed discussion of the item analysis, see Thomas and Ring (1981).

Few studies based on the HMS have been reported, and most of these have been based on small and often ill-defined samples. Table 6.5 presents a comparison of mean scores from the present study with those from all other reported studies. Section VII of the HMS is included, and it is assumed that each respondent in the present study, by virtue of having a hearing loss in excess of 60 dB, would not have normal hearing, thus a score of 3 is scored for that item in Section VII. It is clear, in comparison with most of the other studies, that those in the present study are heavily handicapped. Comparison with findings based on the pilot study is especially interesting. At the piloting stage, the HMS was administered to a group of adults who had suffered severe sensorineural hearing loss (mean = 73 dB) for some time, and were known to have experienced considerable difficulties in coping with the disability. The degree of hearing hand-

TABLE 6.6

Correlations between Hearing Loss Variables[a]

|                        | Mean dB loss | % phonemes (Boothroyd) | SPIN HP[b] | SPIN LP[c] |
|------------------------|--------------|------------------------|------------|------------|
| % phonemes (Boothroyd) | $-0.57^d$    | —                      | —          | —          |
| SPIN HP[b]             | $-0.44^d$    | $0.63^d$               | —          | —          |
| SPIN LP[c]             | $-.036^d$    | $0.64^d$               | $0.85^d$   | —          |
| HMS total score        | $0.08$       | $0.31^d$               | $0.42^d$   | $-0.45^d$  |

[a]$N$ varies between 81 and 88.
[b]HP = high probability condition.
[c]LP = low probability condition.
[d]$p < .05$.

icap in both these groups is remarkably similar. The only other study which found similar levels of hearing handicap is the one reported by Stephens (1980). It is difficult to gauge to what extent Stephens's sample is really comparable. The HMS was administered "to patients being seen in the General Hearing Aid Centre for hearing aid fitting following a consultation in one of the ENT clinics of the Hospital." It is highly likely, therefore, that the majority of patients in Stephens's sample had only just learned that their hearing loss could not be treated. They were about to be fitted with a hearing aid without knowing how effective it would prove to be. By contrast, the respondents in the present study had owned a hearing aid for a minimum of a year. They therefore had had a reasonable time to adjust to the knowledge that their hearing loss could not be treated, and to become accustomed to wearing a hearing aid. Moreover, Stephens did not provide data on either the degree and type of hearing loss, or on the age and sex structure of his sample.

Table 6.6 gives the correlations between HMS, dB loss, and the speech discrimination tests. All the correlations are in the predicted direction except for that between the HMS score and mean dB loss, which is close to zero. The HMS does correlate reasonably well with the speech scores, however. It seems, therefore, that Noble is correct in his contention that hearing for pure tones is a very poor measure of handicap, as subjectively perceived by hearing-impaired people themselves (Noble, 1978).

## IV. EFFECT OF HEARING LOSS ON THE FAMILY[1]

There is a dearth of baseline psychological research on the family *qua* family, that is, where the family is focussed upon as the entity, and concern is with processes of interaction within the family (SSRC, 1981). This probably has much to do with the difficulty of deciding on an appropriate methodology for the study of such a complex phenomenon; as Hinde (1978) put it, the study of interpersonal relationships is still "in quest of a science." It is hardly surprising, therefore, that little is known about the effect of disability on family life (Topliss, 1979). The few reported studies have concentrated on immediate reaction to disability in which onset is almost always traumatic, and in which the family aspect is confined to the husband/wife relationship (cf. Fink *et al.,* 1968; Malone, 1969; Carpenter, 1974; Miles, 1979).

One of the few studies of family response to disability was reported by Cogswell (1976). This was a major study, in which interviews were conducted with all family members over a number of years following the onset of disability. Cogswell recognised the difficulty of assaying family reactions to disability within a comprehensive framework. She attempted to organise the data arising from her open-ended interviews in terms of general sociological theory, general systems theory, and inexplicably, "the arts—a play and a film." Most of her report, however, is devoted to methodological considerations, and to describing a film about a black family coping with impoverishment in the Deep South, a situation she sees as analogous to being physically disabled. Disappointingly, there is no detailed analysis of the interview transcripts within the theoretical framework, which would have made the study useful for comparison purposes.

It will be recalled from the First Study that although hearing loss was associated with psychological disturbance, there was no obvious adverse effect on family life. The proportion of separated/divorced respondents was similar to that found in the general population. Hearing-impaired people were not more likely to have rows about various aspects of married life. They did not spend less time in activities with their children. However, the aspects of family life covered in the First Study could hardly be

[1]This section was written with Margaret Lamont and Margaret Harris.

described as exhaustive. Moreover, there was reason to believe that, despite what has just been said, hearing loss did have an adverse effect on family life. In the first place, although members of the hearing-impaired sample in the First Study were not more likely to have general rows, having rows about deafness stood out prominently, though, of course, this item could not be controlled in a general population study. Secondly, those who believed that hearing loss had affected their families and married lives were more likely to be psychologically disturbed.

In the Second Study, the proportion of the sample who were separated/divorced was very high, indicating that severe sensorineural hearing loss may be related to considerable family stress. In the self-completion questionnaire, respondents were also invited to say how hearing loss had affected relationships with family and friends. The following examples illustrate the very wide range of family difficulties seen from the hearing-impaired person's point of view.

> Question: How has your hearing loss affected your relationship with your family and
> friends?
> 1. It does; cannot hear what they are talking about.
> 2. No, but difficult to join in with chatter of young children. Also difficult to converse
>    with people in other rooms in the house.
> 3. Sometimes I feel very cutoff, as they will not repeat what has been said. This makes
>    things very difficult, and can cause a lot of unhappiness.
> 4. Family—yes. As they could not come to terms with it—but not at all with friends.
> 5. No different than if I had full hearing, except that I cannot be as helpful to them as I
>    could with full hearing.
> 6. By limiting conversational intercourse.
> 7. Family. It can cause irritation, especially when they are tired. Most of my friends
>    are very tolerant.
> 8. My mother gets irritated with me.
> 9. It makes things more difficult for them, but they put up with it.
> 10. It's a tremendous strain on other people to cope with someone who can't hear
>     normally.
> 11. Forty percent responsible for my marriage breakup.
> 12. I think it is only because of the understanding of my family, particularly my
>     husband, that I have managed to live with this loss of hearing. All friends very kind,
>     too.
> 13. No; but wife gets a bit irritable.
> 14. Very difficult to enter into conversation going on within family, Marital relationship
>     strained.
> 15. My relationship is as before my hearing loss.
> 16. Has promoted greater understanding of problems of deaf people, and brought out
>     their (normal hearing people's) sympathy and willingness to be helpful.

17. Not much with family, but with some friends, they get annoyed if I don't hear all they say.
18. Has not made any difference; they just adapt themselves to speak louder.
19. They get impatient with one—but family otherwise sympathetic.
20. Not a great deal, and not to any lasting degree.
21. They feel I don't know what they're talking about, and often they don't have the time or patience to keep repeating words and statements to me.
22. My husband is getting impatient; more difficulties in making friendships.
23. We have all adjusted.
24. Very difficult, but they try to understand.

Taking the above considerations into account we decided to undertake a family study by conducting unstructured, open-ended interviews with respondents, along with any family members (or friends) they chose to be present. Such an approach, it was believed, would be especially useful in providing insights into perspectives of normally hearing people who had to cope with a hearing-impaired family member or close friend. Moreover, it would cater to the very wide range of situations and coping strategies which were expected. Interviewing was carried out in the spring of 1980.

## A. Families

The 27 respondents who agreed to take part in the Family Study differed from the rest of the sample of 88 in two ways. Firstly, they were less likely to be widowed, separated, or divorced (11% compared with 23%), but this was not surprising because, by definition, a "family" study does not include people who live alone. Secondly, they were less likely to be psychologically disturbed (8% compared with 23%). It is likely, therefore, that those families who agreed to be interviewed were relatively well-adjusted and stable. In fact, we noted that a few of those who refused a family interview gave domestic problems as their reason. Table 6.7 shows some of the characteristics of the family sample. Although there was a wide range of hearing loss among the respondents,[2] we found that there was little relationship between the severity of a respondent's hearing loss and the problems experienced by the family.

[2]The term *respondent* is used throughout this chapter to refer to the hearing-impaired individual, as opposed to family and friends who took part in the study.

TABLE 6.7

Characteristics of the Family Sample

A. *Marital Status and Sex of Respondent*

| | Male | Female | Total |
|---|---|---|---|
| Married | 13 | 7 | 20 |
| Single | 2 | 2 | 4 |
| Divorced/separated/widowed | — | 3 | 3 |
| Total | 15 | 12 | 27 |

B. *Age*

| ≤39 | 40–49 | 50–59 | 60–64[a] |
|---|---|---|---|
| 2 | 7 | 12 | 6 |

C. *Social Class*

| I and II (professional) | III (nonmanual) | III (manual skilled) | IV and V (semiskilled/ unskilled) |
|---|---|---|---|
| 7 | 6 | 7 | 7 |

D. *Hearing Loss in Better Ear*[b]

| 60–69 dB | 70–89 | 90+ |
|---|---|---|
| 12 | 8 | 7 |

E. *Family Members Present at the Interview (in Addition to the Hearing-Impaired Respondent)*[c]

| | |
|---|---|
| Spouse | 18 |
| Child/children | 15 |
| Friend | 5 |
| Other relative(s) | 11 |

[a]Males only; Women are not included in the 60–64 age group because they reach retirement age at 60.

[b]Mean of 0.5, 1, 2, and 4 kHz.

[c]In nine interviews, one person only was present in addition to the respondent; in 11 interviews, two persons were interviewed with the respondent; and in six interviews, there were three or more interviewees in addition to the respondent.

The following section will describe the strategies used by families in their attempts to adapt to hearing loss, and then will consider the emotional implications.

## B. Adapting to Hearing Loss

### 1. *Communication*

Nearly all the respondents relied on lipreading at home. Some family members took this into account by ensuring they attracted respondents' attention before starting to speak. Others arranged quite formal, face-to-face family conversations on a regular basis. For example, one couple set aside time to do this each day when they came home from work. A single mother described how she and her teenage children used to sit around a table once a week to "iron out" any problems or misunderstandings. Several families described the methods they used for attracting respondents' attention, including whistling, tapping arms, pulling sleeves, and changing their voice tone.

A few family members used a form of signing to communicate with respondents. A husband described how he used finger spelling to communicate from a distance with his hearing-impaired wife in crowded, noisy places, such as pubs. Another respondent did not use her hearing aid when she was at home alone with her sister—they communicated over whole weekends using their own version of signing.

### 2. *Use of Household Equipment and Environmental Aids*

A variety of aids is available to help the hearing impaired use televisions, telephones, doorbells, alarm clocks, and baby alarms for young infants. In the First Study, the extent of ownership of such environmental aids was found to be very low. Out of a sample of 211 hearing aid owners with all types and degrees of hearing loss, 25 had a telephone aid, two a television aid, three a doorbell aid, and two an alarm clock aid. This low ownership was echoed even in the severely hearing-impaired respondents of the Family Study. In addition, we found that ownership was not necessarily indicative of either usage or benefit (Harris *et al.*, 1981). Of the 27 respondents, three had tried out television aids, but none were being used, only one of four owners of special telephone bells found them useful, four respondents used amplifiers to help them with telephone conversations, five respondents used doorbell aids, and only one had used a special vibrating alarm clock. But there was considerable evidence that this low level of ownership of available environmental aids did not imply any lack of "need" for such aids.

Twenty-four of the 27 respondents had either reluctantly given up watching television or persisted in spite of many difficulties. Ten respondents had the television on so loud that it disturbed other members of the household and/or neighbours. The wife of one respondent said she was glad to have moved recently to a detached bungalow where the noise of the television could not bother the neighbours. The normally hearing son of one woman grew up accustomed to so much noise from the television that he had not outgrown the habit of having the volume "far too loud" even now that he had his own home away from his mother. One young male respondent shared a flat with a student friend. Because he needed to have the television volume turned very high, his student friend had to move to another room and occupy himself in a routine activity such as copying notes. His friend also played music so that the sound of the television did not disturb him.

Apart from the need to have the television on very loud, several respondents disturbed the television viewing of their households in other ways. Four needed a complete absence of background noise in the room. One man's teenage children, for example, said they did not mind their father having the television on very loud but were annoyed at being forbidden to chat to each other in the only living room. Another respondent described how he had to have the sound "just right" when he watched the television news, and that if his wife and daughter talked at all it was "hopeless." Ten respondents relied heavily on their families to help them out when they "lost the thread," to give occasional summaries, or to repeat the "punchline" of jokes. Some family members said that they themselves often missed parts of the programmes, ends of jokes, and suchlike, because they were busy trying to explain previous material to the respondents.

Fifteen of the 27 respondents could not be relied upon to hear the telephone bell, and depended on other members of the household to answer. Therefore, they were vulnerable when left alone. Some respondents regularly used a friend or spouse to make and receive telephone calls. One profoundly deaf respondent had had her own telephone disconnected, and relied on her next-door neighbour to make and receive all calls on her behalf.

Seventeen of the 27 respondents could not normally hear the doorbell. Some had made little or no attempt to solve the problem, while others had evolved a variety of coping strategies, the most obvious and frequent of which was to rely upon other members of the family or household. This also diverted the possible difficulty of having to talk to a stranger on the doorstep. When the hearing-impaired person was alone, however, the problem remained unsolved and could be serious in an emergency. Other methods of coping included sitting at the window to watch for visitors, relying on dogs to bark, and expecting visitors to attract the respondents' attention through the window.

For those caring for babies or invalids, a visual alarm system is available in which a microphone is connected to a warning light. We found two examples of situations in which such an aid would have been very useful. One respondent had shared a bedroom with her ill mother, who put the light on if she needed to attract her hearing-impaired daughter's attention during the night. During the day, the respondent used to time herself to check on her mother every 20 minutes, because she could not hear her calling. Another respondent who was a parent had to check on his young children at frequent intervals during the evening when his wife was out.

Waking up on time is clearly of great importance, especially for those in employment, as were 18 of the respondents. However, only one respondent, a single parent responsible for two teenage children, had an aid, a vibrating alarm. Another respondent's method of waking must be regarded as unsatisfactory for both himself and his wife. He relied on his wife to wake him for work even though this meant she had to wake up one and a half hours earlier than was really necessary for her.

Many respondents were distressed or irritated by the excessive noise generated by televisions, radios, and record players used by other members of their households, and constantly required volumes to be lowered. Some families mentioned that the discomfort felt by the hearing-impaired person seemed to be out of proportion to the "real" volume as perceived by normally hearing persons, especially as the complainants had a hearing loss! The phenomenon of recruitment, responsible for this problem, is discussed on page 13.

Thus, while many hearing-impaired people and their families had developed their own coping strategies, these often placed heavy demands on hearing members of the households. Relying heavily on other members of the family also meant that the hearing-impaired person was vulnerable when left alone.

## 3. *Acting as Intermediaries*

In most group situations, especially those involving strangers, hearing-impaired individuals experience great difficulty. In such situations, families were often particularly supportive. Strategies used to help respondents included "filling in" in group conversations when respondents did not realise they were being spoken to. One husband, for example, always had "half an eye" on his hearing-impaired wife in groups, and intervened if necessary. One wife said that if her husband tried to "opt out" in social situations, she "wouldn't let him get away with it," instead summarising what was being said. Another wife put her husband "on the right track" if he misheard. One respondent's flatmate rephrased group conversations for him in such a way that nobody noticed, and he always arranged to sit on his hearing aid side if they were in a public place. Another respondent could not attend social gatherings without his wife, because he relied on lipreading conversation "clues" from her; when necessary, she asked people to speak more clearly to him. A teenage daughter explained how she sat with her father at church meetings and passed him notes on important topics. Several spouses said they sometimes explained the respondents' hearing loss to strangers, and if necessary, would ask them to speak clearly, or not to shout. One wife always used the term "hard-of-hearing" (she never said "deaf"). One 9-year-old daughter takes over from her father as intermediary for her hearing-impaired mother when the family is on holiday in Germany; the daughter speaks German and the father does not.

There were many examples of families or close friends who helped in dealing with officials, shopkeepers, teachers, etc. One hearing-impaired respondent always took his wife or friend with him to the garage because the people there "couldn't be bothered to speak clearly." The wife of another respondent left him to deal with shop assistants, bus conductors, and so one, but intervened if she felt he was having difficulties. In another family, children remembered that they always used to speak for their mother in shops or explain to strangers that she was "a bit Mutt'un."[3] In two cases, respondents felt unable to cope with shopping, and this was done entirely by their spouses. Such help, however, could be unwelcome; two people said their spouses were sometimes "overprotective" and "took over" in situations where they could have coped on their own. Indeed, in some of our interviews, a hearing member of the family seemed to "take over"completely.

## C. Emotional Implications

### 1. *Stress*

The difficulty of trying to communicate with a hearing-impaired person often gave rise to irritation or impatience. People sometimes gave up in their attempts to communicate, especially if they were feeling tired. One wife often turned on the radio after failing to make herself understood. Another found communicating with her husband so exhausting that she had gradually come to restrict herself to essential communication only; she also found it irritating that when she was out and her husband was at home, she could not telephone him, nor could she rely on him to let her into the house. A few people, however, said they never felt irritated by having to repeat things; one wife said that if she was feeling tired and became impatient, she always apologised afterwards.

There were problems other than those of communication that caused irritation or anxiety in families. At one interview, a wife and daughter said they were irritated by the respondent's constant humming; the respondent said "it helps the loneliness." The family of another respondent complained that she was "very noisy about the house, banging saucepans, etc.," obviously unaware of the noise she was making. Two people were irritated when their spouse affected to hear, one of whom said, "he gets that look on his face and he laughs, and then I know he is pretending"; she also felt that her husband sometimes used his deafness as an excuse to avoid answering her. Another wife complained that sometimes she had to "take over" when they were entertaining because her husband, who did not enjoy "social chitchat," tended to use his hearing as an excuse to

[3]That is, the comic characters Mutt and Jeff. Use of their names here is Cockney rhyming slang for "deaf."

withdraw from the conversation. Three other wives mentioned that they were sometimes hurt on their husbands' behalf by the insensitivity of outsiders who showed signs of impatience, excluded their husbands from conversations, treated them as "deaf and daft," or talked to them through an intermediary. (Ironically, this latter reaction, the "does-he-take-sugar?" phenomenon, may sometimes be *necessary* when strangers are trying to communicate with the hearing impaired.) Another wife worried about her husband's safety when crossing roads if he was out alone. Indeed, only one person seemed to be entirely unaffected by his spouse's hearing loss; he had not even noticed she was losing her hearing until friends and relatives remarked on it; as he put it, "I'm not the affectable type."

We have already mentioned the heavy demands made on family members by the many respondents who had difficulties with television, telephones, and doorbells. Although it is not possible to estimate the extent to which these demands gave rise to stress, it is certain that such dependence could have been substantially reduced by the use of appropriate aids.

Some of the older children talked about earlier days, and there were a number of cases where children had been or still were unhelpful, irritable, or unsympathetic towards their hearing-impaired parent. Mostly these attitudes found expression in "playing up" by younger children, and in failure to speak clearly by older children. For instance, one wife recalled that they went through a "bad period" when their now-teenage son was about 6 years old. He refused to speak clearly and directly to his father, and made *sotto voce* impertinent comments to and about him. An adult brother and sister admitted that, as children, they used to mumble or whisper together, knowing that their mother could not hear them. In some families, unhelpful attitudes appeared to persist into adulthood, although they were no longer so deliberate. One son, for example, said that his mother had been very deaf ever since he could remember, and he had exaggerated her difficulty by speaking softly on purpose. Now in his early 20s, he still became irritable when she could not hear him the first time he said something. He also sometimes forgot to speak clearly to her.

Apart from deliberate provocation, there were other examples of unsympathetic behaviour in children. A father commented that his teenage son became impatient if asked to repeat something, and said "forget it." An adult daughter said she was sometimes very impatient with her mother, particularly in the morning; her mother wakes her up before putting on her hearing aid, and therefore cannot hear what her daughter says. In two other interviews, it emerged that teenage children sometimes shouted to their parent from another room, although they knew they could not be heard. One man mentioned that he had two sons who left home before he became deaf; they had never learned to speak clearly to him, and he could not hear them as well as he could hear his wife and daughter, who lived with him. In this case, it was the father, rather than his sons, who got impatient. Another man's teenage children were very irritated because their father needed complete silence when watching television, and could not tolerate the loud playing of records.

Embarrassment about the respondents' hearing loss was not mentioned by adults, although in several families, where the respondents' effective hearing had been greatly improved by an aid, there appeared to be a reluctance to discuss what life had been like previously. Children, on the other hand were more explicit about embarrassment experienced by themselves or their friends. One 9-year-old daughter, when talking to her schoolfriend, said she wished her mother could hear normally. A teenage daughter in another interview said that when she phones her mother from work, she positions herself so that people cannot see who it is shouting. Two other children mentioned how concerned they were when their parents had to visit their schools and speak to their teachers; they worried that the teachers would not speak clearly, or that their parents might appear foolish.

In six interviews, children mentioned that their friends were embarrassed or uneasy in the presence of the deaf parent. A teenage daughter, for example, said that a few of her friends seemed to feel embarrassed at having to talk loudly, and tended to speak to her so that she could relay the message to her father. The 9-year-old daughter mentioned previously had a friend of 11 years who found it difficult to make her mother understand, and this mother confirmed that her daughter's friends seemed to be shy of her. In another interview, a son thought that his friends understood his mother's deafness, but the mother herself did not agree; she thought that her son's friends were not only embarrassed, but also tended to regard her as stupid, always speaking to her through an intermediary. One man, whose children's friends were embarrassed to meet him, said he could not communicate with them because their voices were unfamiliar. It seems this embarrassment among children may partly be caused by the need to shout, since many people regard shouting as "rude." This point was illustrated by a daughter-in-law who was naturally shy and had a soft voice. She did not feel she could justify shouting unless she had something important to say, so she avoided talking to her father-in-law. Perhaps children are even more self-conscious than adults about having to talk in a special way.

There were also difficulties in communication between deaf parents and their own children. One man said his teenage daughter tended to talk loudly and then he could not hear what she was saying and had to ask his wife to "interpret." One woman said that, as a single parent, deafness had added to her problems in dealing with young children. She had had to be extra-alert to dangers and breaches of discipline, and consequently became very irritable and strict. She had often thought that the children were being cheeky, quarrelling, or plotting against her, and had punished them, only to find later that she had completely misunderstood the situation. A 12-year-old mentioned that he could not have a "good talk with his dad," as other boys could.

Some of these examples illustrate how hearing-impaired parents and children may feel isolated from each other. Three respondents also mentioned how their deafness sometimes excluded them from the relationship between their children and the hearing parent. For example, one man described feeling "very excluded" when his wife and son were talking together. Another could not hear if his wife and daughter were talking together in normal voices, and imagined they were talking about him or being secretive. Upon enquiring into the subject of conversation, he usually found it was of no interest to him.

## 2. *Curtailment of Activities*

As their hearing deteriorated, many respondents had had to discontinue activities and interests such as visits to the theatre, cinema, and pub, going to parties, and attending classes; and usually the spouse was similarly affected. One man, discussing social life, felt that he had suffered more from his wife's deafness than she had herself. In seven families, both the respondent and spouse had curtailed visits to the cinema and/or theatre. Two normally hearing wives had stopped going to classes because they did not wish to go alone. Another hearing wife no longer went to the pub because she could not chat to her husband in the noisy atmosphere. One respondent had stopped taking his wife for drives because he found driving such a strain. The wife of another respondent had decided they should no longer take holidays abroad, in case air travel aggravated her husband's hearing loss. Another respondent could not tolerate the noise in the ballroom at their holiday camp, so he, his wife, and their children had left after a short while each evening.

As described earlier, television viewing was affected in nearly all cases by the need for very loud volume or complete background silence, or by requests to other members of the family to "fill in" for them.

### 3. *Support from the Family*

A number of studies have shown how important it is for disabled people to acknowledge their handicap openly if they are to overcome social discomfort. Comer and Piliavin (1972) have shown how physical disability impairs discourse; Hastorf *et al.* (1979) have demonstrated the importance of acknowledging disability. In the light of this, it is of interest that three families helped respondents by encouraging them not to hide their disability, but to admit to a hearing problem and insist on clear speech from others. One man said that his flatmate's encouragement to do this had been "a turning point in [his] life," and he now felt he could be frank about his hearing if he wished. One wife had managed to persuade her husband to tell his teacher at evening classes about his hearing loss, with the result that the teacher had been most helpful. Another respondent's adult daughter had given her a "talking to" on this subject, and this had made her change her behaviour and be unafraid of admitting her hearing loss. Since then, she had had far fewer problems with shop assistants, ticket clerks, and other strangers.

In three cases, the supportive role of the family was made explicit. One respondent said, "Without my family and friends, I could not manage"; another, that deafness was "not too much of a problem if you have a caring family and friends." Another family felt that if there was "genuine affection in the family," the handicap was reduced to "a nuisance, only."

### D. Conclusion

We suggested that there was reason to believe that the families that participated in this study were relatively well-adjusted. Nevertheless, there was considerable evidence of stress, both for the respondent and for normally hearing members of his or her family. Much of the stress experienced by the respondents appears to have been alleviated by their supportive families, though giving such support could be a source of stress for the nonhandicapped family members.

A rather unexpected finding was the part that suitable environmental aids might have played in improving the quality of life of the whole family. While we knew that such aids were underused by hearing-impaired people in general, we did not expect so few aids to be owned by this severely impaired group, nor that those few aids which were owned would be inappropriate or underused.

On the basis of the findings of the Family Study, there seems to be a strong case for family counselling to be initiated when a hearing aid is first issued. At the same time, it is important that patients be fully acquainted with environmental aids and instructed in their use. Initiating contact when the hearing aid is first issued appears extremely important to us, because this is the time when both the hearing-impaired individual and his or her family are most likely to be receptive to advice and guidance, and therefore most open to counselling.


## V. EMPLOYMENT[4]


In the First Study, the proportion of unemployed respondents was similar to that found in the general population. Similar comparisons with a control group gave no indication of underemployment, insofar as respondents felt that their present job was "about right" for their abilities. Promotion prospects appeared unaffected. However, respondents did worry about work, and were less happy at work. When those in the "severely hearing-impaired" subsample were examined separately, there was still no evidence of unemployment. In comparison with the rest of the hearing-impaired sample, however, respondents in the sub-sample were significantly more likely to have changed jobs due to hearing loss, to feel they had less likelihood of future promotion, to prefer a less demanding job, to feel that hearing loss had adversely affected their work, and to be less

[4]This section written with Margaret Lamont and Margaret Harris.

TABLE 6.8

Factor Analysis of Work Items Based on 55 Respondents Who Completed the Checklist of Difficulties Experienced at Work[a,b]

| Checklist items | N | Factors and loadings | | | |
|---|---|---|---|---|---|
| | | I | II | III | IV |
| *Section A: Dealing with People Other* | | | | | |
| *Than Colleagues (N = 47[c])* | | | | | |
| 1. Difficulty with the telephone | 41 | — | .36 | — | — |
| 2. Difficulty in coping with the public | 32 | — | .36 | — | — |
| *Section B: Formal Work Relations (N = 26[c])* | | | | | |
| 3. Difficulty in dealing with colleagues | 23 | — | — | .98 | — |
| 4. Difficulty in dealing with supervisor | 19 | — | — | .63 | — |
| *Section C: Job Proficiency (N = 29[c])* | | | | | |
| 5. Difficulty in actually doing the job | 27 | — | — | — | .47 |
| 6. Finding it necessary to alter the job in some way | 11 | .34 | — | — | .47 |
| *Section D: Social Relationships (N = 22[c])* | | | | | |
| 7. Difficulty in making friends at work | 9 | .81 | — | .47 | — |
| 8. Feeling left out at work | 21 | .59 | — | — | — |
| 9. Receiving little respect from colleagues | 8 | .57 | .47 | — | — |
| *Section E: Loss of Status (N = 34[c])* | | | | | |
| 10. Loss of ,promotion | 24 | — | — | — | .57 |
| 11. Loss of job | 10 | — | .60 | — | — |
| 12. Less responsibility at work | 18 | — | .53 | — | .53 |
| 13. Demotion | 5 | — | .65 | — | — |

[a]Sixty-eight people in the sample were working, but only 55 felt that their work and/or job prospects were affected, and therefore completed the checklist.

[b]Loading $\geq$ .30.

[c]$N$ = the number of respondents who checked either or both of the items in the section.

happy at work. Therefore, it was important to investigate, in greater depth, the effect of severe hearing loss at work.

Out of the total sample of 88, 68 were working at the time of interview. Of the 68, 55 indicated that hearing loss had affected their work in some way. These 55 then completed a checklist of specific difficulties encountered at work (Table 6.8). Rather obviously, very many respondents had problems with the telephone, and in dealing with people other than colleagues (Section A). The number who agreed upon items covering difficulties with social relationships (Section B) may be an underestimate, because only those who indicated that their work or job prospects had been affected in some way went on to complete the checklist. The most important finding concerned Section E which showed that exactly half of those working (34 out of 68) had experienced loss of job status, 10 of whom had actually lost jobs due to hearing loss. The proportion who had lost jobs (14%) was similar to the proportion who had changed jobs due to hearing loss in the First Study (16%), though changing jobs and losing jobs may not be comparable. The main points, however, are that half the respondents suffered a downgrading in job status, and that 40% (Section C) had difficulties in actually carrying out their work.

In order to verify the extent to which the five areas described in Table 6.8 actually represented separate areas of difficulty, the items were subjected to a Factor Analysis with varimax rotation. The four emerging factors correspond fairly well with the five areas covered in the checklist. Factor II appears to account for both Sections A and E, suggesting, predictably, that it is those who have to communicate with outsiders who are more likely to suffer loss of status or loss of job.

Of the 20 respondents not working at the time of the interview, only four described themselves as unemployed. Presumbaly, the rest were housewives, or had retired. Only two indicated that hearing loss had adversely affected job status at some time in the past. Hearing loss does not appear to have been a major factor in keeping people out of work.

The Family Study described above provided an unexpected opportunity to test the validity of the employment questionnaire. (See also Thomas *et al.*, 1982.) Examination of the interview transcripts revealed that many hearing-impaired respondents had used the opportunity to explain more fully the effect that hearing loss had at work. The many spontaneous comments made about problems related to work serve to illustrate that a structured questionnaire, although undoubtedly useful as a starting point, throws little light on the complex nature of difficulties hearing-impaired people encounter at work.

Two people who indicated on the checklist that their hearing loss had caused them to lose a job at some time explained how this had happened. One woman, a trained hairdresser, felt she could no longer cope when she became severely deaf. She relied entirely on lipreading, and feared she might misunderstand a client's instructions; she also felt that talking to clients was a part of the job, and she was unable to do this. She had since taken a part-time shampooing job. (The loss of the hairdressing job is ironic in view of the fact that hairdressing is a career recommended for the hearing impaired by the Royal National Institute for the Deaf.) The second person who had lost her job due to hearing loss explained that she left her job as a hospital pharmacy clerk when the vertigo associated with her hearing loss became too difficult to cope with. Although the colleagues at her original job had been helpful and had taken care to speak clearly, she found when she subsequently took a few temporary jobs that people were very unsympathetic about her hearing, and eventually she gave up the idea of working altogether.

Four other respondents were found to have lost a job at some time, although they had not indicated this on the employment questionnaire. This may have been because they interpreted "loss of a job" as meaning "dismissal," whereas in actual fact, they had made the decision themselves. One woman had given up her job as a school meals supervisor 12 years before because she felt she could no longer hear the children; she had not worked since. A man had said on the questionnaire at the first interview that he had been "demoted"; at the second interview, he explained that before he suddenly lost his hearing, he had been a works manager, and had spent about 90% of his time on the telephone or meeting people. Following further deterioration of his hearing, he felt he could not cope and accepted a redundancy payment. He subsequently found a job weighing out and packing chemicals, where he worked alone. Another man, a security officer, had retired early at 62 because he could not communicate on a two-way radio; he also felt that his difficulties had been exacerbated by the impatience of his supervisor. A woman who had been severely hearing impaired when first interviewed had completely lost her hearing when interviewed for the Family Study. She was a nursing sister, and although she had some problems at work, such as answering the telephone and taking blood pressures, she had always managed. After she suddenly and completely lost her hearing, she wished to continue her job. She found she could lip-read the patients, and she asked the other nurses to answer the telephone for her. This arrangement worked well for 2 days, but on the third day the nurses refused to cooperate. She was then transferred to administrative work, which she did not like.

Two respondents who indicated on the questionnaire that they had lost promotion explained what had happened. A cleaner lost the chance of promotion because he was unable to use an ordinary telephone, and he had had to refuse another job which involved the use of a "bleep" system, as well as the telephone. The second respondent had applied for promotion but had been turned down because he could not hear at the interview.

Another two people told us how their hearing loss had precluded them from doing the kind of job they would have preferred, an area not covered in the checklist. One had been a printer for 30 years, until made redundant 3 years previously. Because of his hearing, he did not feel confident enough to find a similar job with another organisation; he now works for the same firm as a technician, a job he does not like. The other was a Post Office engineer. After 3 years, during which he studied for qualifications, he had been told that, because of his hearing loss, he was a liability to his workmates and could even endanger lives in some circumstances. The Post Office had wanted to dismiss him, but due to trade union pressure, he had been given routine office work instead.

Five respondents who indicated that they had problems in relationships with colleagues went into more detail at the family interview. Two men said their mates at work sometimes talked softly on purpose so that they could not hear. One of these respondents said he felt left out at work, and could not "get into the clique." A third man felt that he was left out of conversations at work and could not join in the jokes. Another woman described how her supervisor had sometimes deliberately turned away when he spoke to her or had talked with his pipe in his mouth. An office clerk said her colleagues treated her as though she were "deaf and daft."

On the other hand, colleagues could be helpful. Two respondents said they relied on others to cope with the telephone, if need be. One man said his colleagues always spoke clearly to him, and although they sometimes "took the micky" out of him he did not mind.

Finally, it is often claimed that while hearing-impaired people may not be unemployed, they may nevertheless be underemployed [e.g., Markides et al. (1979)]. This study has made us aware that the concept of under-employment is rather nebulous. We found it almost impossible to disentangle the numerous factors involved. For example, people could be in a job with inferior status because (a) it was genuinely impossible to continue in the favoured job because of hearing loss; (b) they did not have the ability to continue in the favoured job, irrespective of hearing loss; or (c) they had suffered unfair discrimination on the basis of hearing loss. Any research on underemployment would also need to take into account the attitudes of employers and colleagues, as well as those of the hearing-impaired individuals.

# CHAPTER SEVEN

# *Overview and Implications for Rehabilitation*

## I. INTRODUCTION

In this chapter, I would like to discuss the major findings from both studies, and to consider the implications which they have for the rehabilitation of adults with acquired hearing loss. In order to impose some structure on this exercise, I will organise the discussion in the context of a schema (referred to in Chapter 1) which can be applied to most forms of physical and sensory dysfunction (Harris, 1971; Wood, 1980), and which has been adapted for auditory dysfunction by Davis (1983). The schema incorporates four domains of dysfunction: disorder, impairment, disability, and handicap. "Disorder" refers to the actual anatomical or physiological damage that can be seen or inferred, such as an immobilised stapes, a malfunctioning cochlea, or a lesion in the auditory nerve. "Impairment" signifies a reduction in basic functions, the most obvious being a reduction in hearing sensitivity. Phonemic discrimination and sound localisation may also be impaired. "Disability" mainly describes the extent to which speech perception has been affected, and also includes a lessened ability to hear warning signals, background noise, music, and so on. "Handicap" is determined by the extent to which the general well-being and quality of life of the individual have been adversely affected. (This definition of handicap is somewhat different from Davis's.) Handicap can obviously extend to members of the family and other close contacts, and interestingly, so too can disability, when the normally hearing experience difficulty in making themselves understood. In general, the four domains in the schema are

150

sequentially dependent, not only with regard to dysfunction but also rehabilitation. There is little point in treating disorder without expecting a significant improvement in the other domains of hearing dysfunction. Similarly, fitting a hearing aid to reduce impairment will not be of much use unless the ability to hear meaningful sounds is increased; this, in turn, will be of very limited use if improvement does not extend to everyday listening conditions, thereby effectively reducing disability and handicap. If a hearing aid does not adequately compensate impairment and disability, then certain other rehabilitative techniques can be employed, such as auditory training and lipreading tuition, both of which are for the most part located in the disability domain. If treatment and/or rehabilitation within the first three domains is successful, then handicap will be reduced. If not, then residual handicap itself can be alleviated through readjustment, adaptation, change in lifestyle, and so on, and these can be facilitated with appropriate rehabilitative guidance and counselling.

The main focus of the research described in the preceding chapters is on the handicap domain. Before considering the relationship between handicap and the other three domains, it is first of all essential to accept that hearing loss actually does have a sufficiently adverse affect on personal well-being and quality of life to make it a significantly handicapping condition. If people are relatively unaffected by hearing loss, or are able to adapt to a new and satisfactory lifestyle without too much difficulty, with or without the help of a hearing aid, then we would have to conclude that hearing loss is little more than a nuisance. On the other hand, if hearing loss is shown to cause a marked deterioration in psychological well-being, then we must accept that it is a real handicap and proceed to explore the nature of the handicap itself and to relate it to the other three domains of auditory dysfunction. The answer to the question of whether hearing loss is a handicap was quantified with inventories of personality and psychological disorder. The point of using these measures is that they allow one to make an objective decision, based on standardised comparisons with general population norms.

With regard to the effect of acquired hearing loss on personality structure, we can safely conclude that it does not cause increased levels of suspiciousness, does not predispose the individual to a paranoid psychosis, or does not bring about any measurable change in personality whatsoever. Existing evidence in support of a supposed association between hearing loss and paranoid mental states was found to be inadequate when subjected to close scrutiny in Chapter 2. Then, the mild suspiciousness scale included in the First Study failed to differentiate the hearing-impaired sample from the general population sample. Finally, a straightforward personality inventory, the Eysenck Personality questionnaire, did not even discriminate adults with severe to complete hearing loss from population norms. This is the first time that suspiciousness and personality have been investigated in reasonably representative samples of the hearing-impaired population. The only study claiming to detect gross personality disturbance in a hearing-impaired sample rather surprisingly found a substantial number of paranoid schizophrenics in a group of patients on the day before they were to undergo surgery for conductive hearing loss (Maphapatra, 1974a,b). A more rigorous study of the psychiatrically ill population was able to differentiate patients with affective and paranoid psychoses on the basis of hearing losses of 31 and 41 dB, respectively (Kay et al., 1976). To my knowledge, no one has ever reported any behavioural consequences based on such a small difference. These studies, and others, are discussed in more detail in Chapter 2. Studies of the effect of visual impairment and physical disability on personality have also found that basic personality structure remains intact even when disablility is very severe (Shontz, 1970; Keegan et al., 1976). In a recent survey of public attitudes to hearing loss, Bunting (1981) found that "no common stereotype or general picture of deaf people emerged"—hardly likely if the population of adults with acquired hearing loss contained a large number of hypersuspicious individuals, some of whom displayed the symptoms of paranoid psychosis. Incidentally, in a community study of hearing loss among the elderly, my former colleagues Gilhome Herbst and Humphrey (1980) investigated the suggestion that hearing loss of longstanding duration could be related to onset of dementia in old age (Kay et al., 1964; Hodkinson, 1973), and found there was no basis for it. Once again, the belief that hearing loss might be implicated in a fundamental psychological change was unfounded. With regard to rehabilitation, it is essential that all professional staff who come into contact with hearing-impaired people should treat them as normal people who have difficulty in hearing, and attribute any behaviour which, on the surface, appears to be bizarre, to a difficulty in communication, rather than to any presumed psychological abnormality. I hope that the myth dating from 1915 (when Kraepelin reported a single case of a paranoid patient who was hearing-impaired) and which has been incorporated into an official policy statement of the British Society of Audiology (Markides *et al.*, 1979) will now be quietly forgotten.

Although hearing loss does not affect basic personality structure, there is little doubt that a sizeable proportion (at least one in five) of hearing-impaired adults, with whatever type or degree of hearing loss, experience a high level of psychological disturbance long after having acquired a hearing aid and receiving any other form of rehabilitation available at that time. Psychological disturbance is a disorder at the psychoneurotic level and does not result in obviously abnormal behaviour, as is the case with most forms of personality disorder. Essentially, psychological disturbance involves markedly increased levels of stress, which we all experience at some time or another. Typical components of psychological disturbance are anxiety, depression, sleep disturbance, listlessness, panic, and hysteria, from which the majority of people would normally recover spontaneously. It seems, however, that living with hearing loss for a prolonged period may well cause psychological disturbance to become chronic (Janis, 1969). Moreover, the proportion estimated to be psychologically disturbed is probably a very conservative one. In the first place, the inventory used to measure psychological disturbance in both studies has a very severe cutoff point compared with similar inventories (e.g., Goldberg's General Health Questionnaire), and therefore, may not have detected a number of respondents with milder, though still significant, levels of stress. Secondly, it is possible that the proportion identified as disturbed would have been considerably higher at the time of initial attendance at the ENT department, when they would have learned that no treatment was possible and would have been advised to obtain a hearing aid. It is also important to realise that both studies were community-based, rather than hospital-based, and that almost all respondents had kept in contact with the hearing aid clinic only for the replacement of batteries and hearing aid maintenance. Stress associated with hospital attendance would not therefore be a contributory factor.

Having established that hearing loss causes psychological disturbance and is therefore a seriously handicapping condition, it becomes essential to examine the relationship between the other domains of auditory dysfunction and hearing handicap. As was stated above, the four domains are, for the most part, sequentially dependent. Handicap therefore results largely from our inability to intervene successfully in the first three domains. The following discussion will examine what has been learned about the relationship between handicap and the other three domains, and when appropriate, suggestions will be made regarding rehabilitation.

## II. DISORDER; IMPAIRMENT; DISABILITY; HANDICAP

Apart from the simple differential diagnosis between conductive and sensorineural hearing loss, very little is known about hearing disorders. Intervention is almost wholly confined to medical and surgical treatment of middle ear disorders. People with conductive hearing loss that, for some reason, has not been remedied, should not, theoretically, suffer any real impairment, disability, or handicap, because sufficient amplification should restore speech perception to normal, as has been demonstrated under laboratory conditions by Hood and Poole (1971). The real-life situation, in which speech is at a conversational level, usually against a background of noise, is much less satisfactory. Respondents with conductive losses were included in the First Study, and as expected, gained more in terms of speech discrimination from unaided to aided than did respondents with sensorineural losses. However, when performance in the aided condition alone was compared, those with conductive losses were only marginally less disabled. With regard to handicap, respondents with conductive losses were equally likely to be psychologically disturbed. This is rather perplexing, because it should be possible to alleviate much of the disability and handicap due to conductive hearing loss, if not through medical or surgical treatment, then with better hearing aid fitting procedures. If not, then we need to learn why it is that people with apparently remediable disorders are not being adequately rehabilitated. No attempt was made to differentiate within the realm of sensorineural hearing loss in either study; in fact, there appears to be very little known in the disorder domain which could have implications for rehabilitation in any of the other domains of auditory dysfunction.

It seems that we are only beginning to appreciate that the impairment domain of auditory dysfunction is much more complex than was previously thought. Auditory impairment does not simply consist of loss of hearing sensitivity, coupled with distortion caused by frequencies being differentially affected. It is now known, for example, that a number of impairments independently affect the perception of sound (Lutman, 1983). Fundamental research on these aspects of impairment will no doubt lead to an improvement in hearing aid design and to better programmes of behavioural rehabilitation. In the foreseeable future, however, it seems that auditory sensitivity, as measured by the pure tone audiogram, is going to continue to be the principal index of impairment which will be utilised in programmes of rehabilitation. Unfortunately, apart from gross distinctions (for example, between mild and very severe losses, or between flat and markedly sloping losses), the pure tone audiogram has not been found to be a very useful predictor of disability or handicap. In the First Study, it was only minimally related to believing oneself to be a handicapped person, and in the Second Study, a zero correlation was found between dB loss and subjective estimates of hearing disability in the Hearing Measurement Scale. On the other hand, in the First Study, respondents with severe hearing loss (70 + dB) were far more likely to be psychologically disturbed than those with less severe losses. Although this finding was not replicated in the Second Study, in which the majority of respondents had a severe loss, the finding is still more than likely to be a valid one, as it occurred in each of the three hospitals which comprised the sample for the First Study. It is difficult to interpret why the finding was not replicated in the Second Study; a possible explanation is that the sample in the Second Study was drawn largely from one hospital, which may have been atypical. It would obviously be worthwhile to investigate more rigorously the relationship between severe hearing loss and psychological disturbance.

A side effect of auditory dysfunction within the impairment domain is tinnitus, extreme forms of which are known to be highly stressful. The British Tinnitus Association has been formed to offer advice and guidance to people who suffer from the condition, whether or not they have a hearing loss. However, it cannot, by any means, be said that the experience of tinnitus is necessarily stressful, at least if one allows enough time to elapse to come to terms with the condition. In neither study was the experience of tinnitus associated with psychological disturbance or any other handicap variable, a finding confirmed in a recent survey carried out in Australia by Hyde et al. (1981). It does seem that a small minority of tinnitus sufferers do find the condition very upsetting, as was found to be the case in the Second Study, in which respondents were actually asked if it upset them. This was also found to be so in the National Study of Hearing (Davis, 1983). However, it is important not to allow mistaken expectations to lead to inappropriate rehabilitation. Reported tinnitus is not necessarily stressful, and care should be taken not to create a stressful situation out of a nuisance, and possibly, to recommend treatment which has a limited chance of success, and which may, in the case of drug prescription, result in unwanted side effects. It goes without saying that if patients themselves report a great deal of stress due to tinnitus, they should be taken very seriously, and the condition taken into account in the formulation of the individual's rehabilitation programme.

Before moving on to the domains of disability and handicap, I would like to consider onset and progression of hearing loss, both of which are probably relevant to all four domains of auditory dysfunction. A better understanding of these variables should assist in differential diagnosis of auditory disorder and impairment, and would almost certainly contribute to a better understanding of disability and handicap. Obtaining reliable data on onset and progression of hearing loss is another matter, as was amply illustrated in both studies. One of the problems appears to be that onset can be defined differently, according to which domain of auditory dysfunction is being considered. It must be almost impossible, given that onset is usually extremely gradual, to date the actual appearance of the disorder, especially as it will have no noticeable effect on any of the other domains. Perhaps this is why a number of respondents, in an effort to provide a concrete answer about onset of hearing loss, seemed to turn to any ear problem they had previously experienced, often referring to disorders, presumably middle ear ones, experienced in childhood. There is, of course, no known connection between such disorders and the onset of sensorineural hearing loss in later life. Other respondents attempted to pinpoint the time when loss of hearing sensitivity became noticeable. Given that hearing loss needs to be considerable before it has a noticeable effect, such information will be of little use in determining the time of onset of the disorder. Also, hearing loss will not necessarily become an impairment, disability, or handicap as soon as it becomes noticeable. The same, presumably, applies to the onset of other impairments, such as speech distortion. It therefore seems unlikely that any useful information about the onset of hearing disorders or impairments will be obtained by direct questioning of the kind used in the two studies. It is plain that other methods need to be used, longitudinal general population studies for example.

It is hardly surprising that onset, as it is usually measured, contributes little to our understanding of the effects of hearing loss in the domains of disability and handicap. In fact, the only reliable conclusion is that many people wait an inordinately long time following onset of hearing loss before acquiring a hearing aid, a finding confirmed by many others (e.g., Brooks, 1981; Hyde *et al.*, 1981). It is unlikely that there is a simple explanation for this and presumably, several factors are involved. A reason often given is that general practitioners are sometimes reluctant to refer patients who report hearing loss to a hospital consultant when it seems to him or her that the patient does not really have a problem. Few patients will experience much difficulty in a one-to-one conversation in the quiet of the doctor's office, especially because as a great deal of the conversation will be rather predictable. In a study of the elderly hearing impaired, Humphrey *et al.* (1981) found that doctors failed to refer a substantial number of hearing-impaired patients for specialist examination, and extreme cases apart, there is no reason to expect they will be any less reluctant to refer younger patients of employment age. Other reasons why patients wait so long before obtaining a hearing aid probably include resistance to wearing a hearing aid, reluctance to give in to what is seen as part of the ageing process, tolerance of disability, fear of stigma, and so on.

Two other points about onset and progression are worth mentioning briefly. Firstly, with a few exceptions, there was very little or no deterioration in hearing in the years following the acquisition of a hearing aid (between 1 and 7 years). This reinforces the view that onset is so gradual that it may well go unnoticed for a very long time. It could also help to explain why many respondents in the First Study, in which the majority had mild or moderate losses, did not appear to connect reduction in psychological well-being with hearing loss, possibly attributing it to other causes, such as an inevitable deterioration in the quality of life associated with ageing. Secondly, not one of the respondents in the Second Study who reported that onset had been sudden was psychologically disturbed. There is possibly some truth in the belief that it is easier to come to terms with a sudden, if traumatic, disability than to suffer the uncertainty associated with gradual onset.

A great deal more research needs to be done across the four domains of auditory dysfunction if we are to obtain a better understanding of the factors governing onset and progression of hearing loss. Insofar as rehabilitation is concerned, it is much more important to obtain a detailed account of progression of hearing loss than it is to attempt to establish date of onset, which in most, though not all, cases will have dubious validity, and little or no significance. What I mean by ''progression'' is much more than shifts in loss of sensitivity or in deterioration in speech discriminability. If rehabilitation is to be geared to individual needs, then ''progression'' has to be defined in psychosocial terms, dealing with changes in relationships within the life sphere of the individual. Careful and sensitive interviewing techniques need to be developed, especially if critical changes are to be identified, and if the effects of hearing loss on a person's life are to be fully understood.

The most interesting finding concerning the relationship between the domains of disability and handicap was the relationship between speech discrimination and psychological disturbance. When the relationship was discovered in the First Study, I naturally assumed that psychological disturbance was the dependent variable, and that it occurred as a consequence of stress associated with a decreasing ability to understand speech and to communicate effectively. However, while the finding was confirmed in the Second Study, it was confined to the speech test, which had also been used in the First Study (Boothroyd Word Lists), failed to generalise to another speech test (the SPIN Test), and was unrelated to subjective estimates of ability to hear speech. Why this should be is difficult to explain, especially if one accepts that hearing for single words in isolation, as with the Boothroyd Word Lists, is far less indicative of communicative ability than hearing for words in context, as in the SPIN Test, or of subjective estimates of communicative ability in real-life situations. A possible explanation, and one for which there is empirical support, is that certain aspects of psychological disturbance affect speech discrimination of single words, rather than the other way around; in other words, it could be that psychological disturbance is the independent, rather than the dependent, variable. The evidence supporting this explanation derives from a study by Malone and Hemsley (1977), in which normally hearing, depressed adults were shown to experience a decrement in auditory sensitivity, and to adopt a conservative response strategy in a signal detection experiment, that is, one in which stimuli are presented close to threshold. It will be recalled that the measure of psychological disturbance, the SAD, consists of two scales, one of which is depression. For normally hearing, depressed people who rarely have to listen to speech near threshold, reduced sensitivity is unlikely to affect normal communication in any way. However, the further reduction in speech discrimination could be critical for those who already have a hearing impairment, at least, when faced with discriminating single words in the absence of contextual clues. It seems, therefore, that a rehabilitation programme, which addresses itself to the handicap domain of auditory dysfunction and explores ways in which to improve the quality of life of hearing-impaired people, might actually bring about an improvement in speech perception and reduce hearing disability, as well as handicap.

The overall conclusion concerning the speech tests used in both studies is similar to that reached by Noble (1978): They tell us very little about the ability to perceive speech in real-life situations. While the tests correlated reasonably well with each other and with hearing for pure tones, the correlations with self-estimate of hearing loss and with subjective quantification of hearing ability for speech were rather low. It seems, therefore, that speech tests tap a very limited area within the disability domain. This might explain why it was in the First Study that no relationship was found between the speech test and variables within the handicap domain. Speech tests may be very useful in the diagnosis of hearing disorders and impairments, or for identifying specific hearing disabilities which auditory training and tuition in speechreading could aim to remedy. However, a great deal of research needs to be carried out in real-life situations if we really want to know how hearing loss affects speech communication. Noble (1983) discusses this problem in some detail.

All the respondents, in both studies, had possessed a hearing aid for at least a year, and most for a considerably longer period. At the same time, only a minute proportion had received any other form of rehabilitation, such as auditory training, speechreading tuition, or counselling. The research in both studies can be viewed, therefore, as an attempt to measure the effectiveness of the hearing aid in reducing disability and handicap. With regard to reduction of disability, around half the respondents in the First Study obtained little or no benefit from their hearing aids, as quantified by the gain between unaided and aided speech discrimination of monosyllabic words presented singly. Those who did benefit most from their hearing aids were not less likely to be psychologically disturbed, or to experience any other measureable reduction in psychological or psycho-social well-being. If we take the amount of time that a hearing aid is used to indicate benefit, we get little further. Reported daily usage of hearing aids, while related to degree of impairment in terms of severity of loss, was unrelated to any aspect of disability or handicap, even to gain in speech discrimination. Thus, it seems that while the hearing aid must obviously be of considerable benefit to a substantial proportion of users, we still do not know how to measure this benefit, or why it is that some people seem to benefit more than others. Above all, we still know very little about hearing aid benefit in everyday situations, a view shared by Kapteyn (1977), who argues that different criteria of satisfaction with hearing aids may apply to different subgroups of the hearing-impaired population. It is clear that research aimed at understanding better just what hearing aid benefit is will have to move out of the hearing aid clinic and into the real world. The part played by environmental aids in the alleviation of disability and handicap will be discussed below, in the context of the Family Study.

It must be obvious from the preceding analysis that most of what is known about the first three domains of auditory dysfunction contributes very little to our understanding of the nature of the handicap which the hearing-impaired person is likely to experience in everyday life. The high incidence of psychological disturbance indicates the severity of the hand-icap, which is at least as severe as the handicap resulting from physical disability (see Chapter 4). However, this still does not tell us how living with hearing loss makes people psychologically disturbed. In this respect, the inventory of psychological disturbance is somewhat analogous to the pure tone audiogram, which points to the likelihood of a communication problem, but is not a very useful indicator of communication difficulties. If we are to reduce psychological disturbance, we obviously need to know much more about psychosocial factors, or what it actually means to live with a hearing loss. In the First Study, the handicap domain was explored by comparing various aspects of the quality of life of hearing-impaired people with general population norms. With regard to employment, re-spondents were no more likely to be out of work than their hearing counter-parts, contrary to popular belief; promotion prospects appeared unaffected, and in general, people felt that the work they were doing was commensurate with their abilities, and that they were not underemployed. Marital status was also unaffected, divorce and separation rates being almost identical to those found in the general population. Moreover, respondents were not more likely to have disagreements about those aspects of married life most likely to be adversely affected by hearing loss. On the other hand, the respondents in the First Study were more likely to be unhappy at work, and many felt that hearing loss had adversely affected their marriages. As a group they were lonely, had fewer friends, and found it more difficult to make friends. They were in poorer general health and were more likely to have a second physical disability or health problem, over and above that of hearing loss, than were members of the control sample. This also applies to adults with physical disabilities (Eastwood and Trevelyan, 1972). It is hardly surprising that the respondents in the First Study were dissatisfied with the overall quality of their lives in comparison with the control sample. From these findings, it seems that hearing loss is associated with a marked deterioration in the quality of life, though not to the extent of causing loss of work or formal marital breakdown. Most surprisingly, none of the measures of the quality of life were related to perceiving oneself to be a handicapped person. Although around half the sample described themselves as "handicapped" people, using the popular meaning of the term, they were indistinguishable from the rest of the sample with regard to all the other variables in the handicap domain, or for that matter, in any of the other domains.

The handicap domain was studied in greater depth in the Second Study, this time confined to adults with severe sensorineural hearing loss. Most people tend to spend a great deal of time at home, and the Family Study, based on a subsample drawn from the sample in the Second Study, attempted to find out how members of the family coped with severe hearing loss, and what the problems were, as perceived by different members of the family. In general, the families interviewed turned out to be very supportive, though this was probably a reflection of the sampling protocol which favoured the participation of "normal" and intact families. Hearing members of the families often acted as intermediaries, or took over responsibility for dealing with outsiders. Sometimes they helped the hearing-impaired person come to terms with hearing loss. Nevertheless, difficulties often arose both within the family, and in contacts with outsiders, many reporting the disrupting effects on communication to be very stressful. A particular area of difficulty concerned children, who were often embarrassed in the presence of outsiders, sometimes took advantage of their parents' hearing loss or acted up, and in some cases were simply unsympathetic. It is not surprising that being supportive was stressful for the hearing spouse or other person on whom family responsibility fell. It is worth stressing again that these families had probably adjusted rather well to hearing loss. In fact, some of those interviewed seemed themselves to be adequate rehabilitators, believing that if there was genuine understanding and affection in the family, the handicap could be reduced to what one described as a "nuisance only." It is likely that coping with a severe hearing loss in those households which did not wish to participate in the Family Study would have been much more difficult, and even worse for those living alone, although the problems of the latter group would probably have been different in nature. What really stood out in the Family Study, however, was the sheer diversity of problems encountered, of communication strategies adopted, and of other methods of coping, even in this relatively homogeneous group (see Chapter 6). The only finding of general applicability concerned the extent to which the acquisition of appropriate environmental aids would almost certainly have resulted in an improvement in the overall quality of life. Time and again, specific problems which families mentioned could have been solved, or partly solved, with such an aid. However, very few possessed environmental aids, and even those that did often found that, for some reason, they did not function satisfactorily, though this did not necessarily mean that there was anything wrong with the aid—it was just not the right one. It is a serious cause for concern that a group of such severely impaired people should not have received direct help in the choice and installation of environmental aids. Benefits which accrue from the time-consuming and labour-intensive procedure of counselling individuals and their families about living with hearing loss may be difficult to quantify and slow to appear. On the other hand, assessment of requirement for environmental aids, even if undertaken in the home, is much more straightforward, and should have an immediate and substantial effect.

With regard to problems encountered at work by respondents in the Second Study, it emerged that about half of those working had experienced loss of status of some kind, and that a sizeable number had, at one time or another, lost their jobs as a direct result of hearing loss. It cannot be said, however, that hearing-impaired people remain out of work, because the rate of unemployment in the sample was found to be the same as in the First Study, that is, equivalent to that found in the general population. Loss of status was found to be associated with communication problems, and with actually doing the work efficiently. Simple remedies, including telephone adaptation, better lighting, or simply moving furniture around, can help improve communication and increase independence, thereby enhancing the status of the hearing-impaired person. Colleagues and supervisors can also be educated to a better understanding of hearing loss. Suggestions such as these are by no means new and have been advocated by various organisations and experts for some time, often being called "hearing tactics" (von der Lieth, 1972a). I believe that if rehabilitation is confined to such measures, it will have a very limited success, simply because the work situation of each individual will almost certainly be unique in a number of respects. This was shown to be the case when the forced-choice, "yes" or "no" answers in the employment problems questionnaire were compared with detailed accounts of what had actually happened in individual cases (see Chapter 6 for examples).

I would now like to turn to the more general implications which the findings in the handicap domain have for rehabilitation. I have already emphasised that personality structure is unaffected by hearing loss, and that hearing-impaired people are not more likely to suffer a paranoid psychosis. They do not even become mildly suspicious. The onus is, therefore, on the rehabilitator to treat the hearing-impaired person as a normal person, with a disability which is likely to prove very stressful and psychologically disturbing. With regard to the high likelihood of psychological disturbance, I would certainly not advocate the routine administration of inventories of psychological disturbance in order to detect those who might need more intensive rehabilitation. Such inventories are useful as research tools, but can be no substitute for detailed knowledge of individual cases. They only point to the likelihood of psychological disturbance, and moreover, have little diagnostic significance (Eastwood, 1971). Neither would I advocate referral to a psychiatrist, except in extreme cases, and I would not expect referral to be any higher than for any other disabled group. It is essential, however, that the person most concerned with rehabilitation should acquire skills in basic psychological assessment, in order to identify those who are under severe stress. Having done so, it is even more important to obtain an insight into the psychosocial lifestyle of each person, in order to find out which aspects of everyday life are causing the most stress. This may not be a simple process by any means, as the Family Study served to show. It also emerged from comments offered spontaneously in the course of the family interviews that the effects of hearing loss at work might be equally complex. It is only through a careful case study approach for each individual that causes of stress can be identified, and a valid distinction made between those who are badly affected by hearing loss and those (a) for whom the hearing aid has reduced disability sufficiently to minimise the consequent handicap to an acceptable level or (b) who have come to terms with, and adjusted to, a significant residual disability to such an extent that they can withdraw from a programme of rehabilitation at a much earlier point than would normally be expected. For those who appear to be psychologically disturbed, the task of finding out which aspects of family, social, or work life are responsible will not be an easy one, partly because of the complex nature of psychosocial life, and also because the very gradual onset of hearing loss which the large majority experience will make it very difficult to disentangle deterioration in the quality of life due to hearing loss from other factors and life events. Also, the finding in the First Study that respondents who felt handicapped by hearing loss were no more likely to be psychologically disturbed than those who did not feel handicapped by hearing loss suggests that many people may not even be aware of the cumulative and insidious effect of the very gradual loss of hearing on the quality of their lives.

If rehabilitation in the handicap domain of auditory dysfunction is to be effective, members of the family and other close contacts and work associates should be involved wherever possible, not only because they are directly affected by impaired communication, but also because they may have different perspectives on what the problems actually are. Then the rehabilitator would be able to obtain a more accurate picture of the whole situation. The decision to include others in the rehabilitation programme should be very carefully considered, of course. It may not be in the best interests of the hearing-impaired individual and could be viewed as an intrusion. It will be recalled that many respondents in the Second Study who were approached to take part in the Family Study declined to do so. Also, Bird and Trevains (1978) found that hearing-impaired clerical workers were resistant to having their disability brought to the attention of

others. On the other hand, of course, many may feel that help from outs
will be beneficial. This was confirmed by a finding in the First Stud
reported by Gilhome Herbst (1980), that many respondents felt membei
of their families did not really understand what it meant to lose one's
hearing. Hyde *et al.* (1981) found that hearing-impaired people, in general,
felt it would be helpful if someone were to explain the effects of hearing
loss to members of their families. Another good reason for taking rehabilitation out of the hearing aid clinic and into the home and place of
work is that it will allow the responsibility for adjusting to the effects of
hearing loss to be shared, and not to fall exclusively on the shoulders of the
impaired person (cf. Noble, 1983). Otherwise, any failure to respond
positively to rehabilitation may be ascribed to the hearing-impaired individual, commonly called "blaming the victim" (for what is a defect in this
community). Finally, if rehabilitation is confined to the hearing aid clinic,
it will be difficult to gauge the practical benefits obtained from the hearing
aid, environmental aids, auditory training, speechreading tuition, and so
one.

The expectation that knowledge about the disorder, impairment, and
disability domains of auditory dysfunction would lead to a better understanding of the nature of hearing handicap has not been fulfilled. Moreover, it does not seem likely that current research in the first three domains
will yield very much information which could be put to practical use for
some time to come (Lutman and Haggard, 1983). For the foreseeable
future, therefore, it seems there will be a large number of hearing-impaired
people with a considerable degree of residual handicap, even after they
have obtained and become accustomed to wearing a hearing aid. It is
therefore essential that much more effort should be expended in finding out
what it means for each individual to live with his or her hearing loss and
what effect it has on those around him or her, so that a rehabilitation
programme can be devised which is tailored to his or her individual needs.
I believe that future research should not be confined to looking for common
problems faced by hearing-impaired people, if only because individual
situations vary so greatly. What is needed now is an action–research
approach, in which the focus is on rehabilitation strategies used to tackle
individual problems, instead of on making generalisations about the kinds
of problems likely to be encountered. The subsequent evaluation of the
extent to which rehabilitation objectives have been achieved then becomes

the research element. This approach has the virtue of combining research with practical application. A better understanding of acquired hearing loss should emerge if individual problems and rehabilitative procedures are documented in detail, and their success (or otherwise) carefully analysed. In other words, research should now become the province of the practitioner and should aim to delineate strategies for reducing the effect of hearing loss on the day-to-day life of those affected.

A final point: Most of what has been written in this book does not apply to people with complete or near-complete hearing loss, although it was originally hoped that a sizable subsample could have been singled out for separate analysis. Even in the Second Study, however, only a handful of respondents could be described as coming into this category. The proportion of adults of at least employment age who have no useful residual hearing is, therefore, extremely small, even within a sample restricted to those with severe hearing loss (cf. Davis and Thornton, 1983). Only through a very large-scale study could such a rare population be adequately sampled. No systematic rehabilitation programme has ever been devised for this tiny group of extremely disabled people, and little is known about the psychological and psychosocial consequences of complete hearing loss, whether onset has been sudden or gradual. It is to be hoped that both the lack of knowledge and the lack of provision will be remedied in the near future.

# First Study: Interview Schedule Used in First Study

Polytechnic of North London  Department of Applied Social Studies 1976
Social and Psychological Implications of
Acquired Deafness for Adults of Employment Age

Name _____     Questionnaire

Address _____        Complete        ☐1

                                    Incomplete      ☐2

Case No. ☐☐☐                        Question numbers: (see notes)


Interviewer        A    ☐1    Type of deafness

                   B    ☐2    sensorineural    ☐1

                   K    ☐3    conductive       ☐2

                   M    ☐4    mixed            ☐3

                        ☐5    other            ☐4


Date of Interview             Tinnitus

                                    none        ☐1

Age                  ☐☐           high pitch     ☐2

                                    low pitch      ☐3

Sex            M    ☐1           other          ☐4

               F    ☐2

                              Personal Disturbance Scale

Year of first appointment  ☐☐   (SAD)              sA   ☐☐

                                                   sD   ☐☐

Length of interview in minutes                     sAD  ☐☐
(excluding audiometry and speech
discrimination)          ☐☐☐
                              Self estimate of deafness

                                    without hearing aid    ☐

                                    with hearing aid       ☐

167

Speech discrimination result

   phonemes  % aided      ☐☐☐

            % unaided    ☐☐☐


<u>dB loss</u>            Hospital

   250 Hz             ☐☐☐

   500 Hz             ☐☐☐

   1 kHz              ☐☐☐

   2 kHz              ☐☐☐

   4 kHz              ☐☐☐

Mean dB loss
(excluding 250 Hz)      ☐☐☐


                  PNL

   250 Hz             ☐☐☐

   500 Hz             ☐☐☐

   1 kHz              ☐☐☐

   2 kHz              ☐☐☐

   4 kHz              ☐☐☐

Mean dB loss
(excluding 250 Hz)      ☐☐☐


Ear tested

                  left       ☐1

                  right      ☐2


Sample source

Time started [          ]

1. I'd like to start our discussion by asking you a few questions about
   your hearing aid and things to do with your hearing in particular.
   Here is a scale. (GIVE CARD A) I'd like you to show me where you
   would place yourself upon it. In other words, where would you first
   say, "Yes, this is me." First of all, all without your aid and then
   when you wear your aid. (CLARIFY WHERE NECESSARY.)

| Can you | Without aid | With aid |
|---|---|---|
| 1. Hear a whispered voice? | 1 | 1 |
| 2. Hear easily in a hall, cinema, or theatre? | 2 | 2 |
| 3. Hear easily in a group, where a few people are chatting together? | 3 | 3 |
| 4. Hear easily someone facing you when they are speaking in a normal voice? | 4 | 4 |
| 5. Hear easily someone facing you when they speak in a loud voice? | 5 | 5 |
| 6. You cannot hear speech at all. | 6 | 6 |

(TAKE BACK CARD A)

2. Could you tell me how old you are?          _____

3. How old were you when you first had trouble with your hearing?

          [  |  ]

3a. Difference between Q. 2 and Q. 3          [  |  ]

4.  Who was it who suggested to you that
    you should do something about it?                    self                        ☐1

                                                          school                      ☐2

                                                          spouse                      ☐3

                                                          family                      ☐4

                                                          paramedical worker          ☐5

                                                          general practitioner        ☐6

                                                          commercial dealer           ☐7

                                                          someone at work             ☐8

                                                          other                       ☐9


5.  And how much time do you think passed
    between feeling you had a hearing loss               immediately                 ☐1
    and going to see your doctor about it?
                                                          less than 3 months          ☐2

                                                          4-6 months                  ☐3

                                                          7-11 months                 ☐4

                                                          1-3 years                   ☐5

                                                          more than 3 years           ☐6

                                                          not applicable (n.a.)       ☐7


6.  Now let's talk about your National Health Service (NHS) aid.
    6a.  What type of NHS hearing aid have you got?

                                           postaural      BE11                       ☐1

                                                          BE12                       ☐2

                                           bodyworn       OL56                       ☐3

                                                          OL58                       ☐4

                                                          OL63                       ☐5

                                                          OL67                       ☐6

                                                          other                      ☐7

                                                          none                       ☐8

6b.  If bodyworn, do you know that a behind-the-
     ear aid is available on the NHS?

                                              yes   ☐1

                                              no    ☐2

7.  People vary in the amount of time they wear
    their hearing aid.  How often do you wear your
    NHS aid?                                 always    ☐1

                                             often     ☐2

                                             sometimes ☐3

                                             rarely    ☐4

                                             never     ☐5

8.  Some people feel that maybe there is not enough
    time spent on explaining how to use their NHS    enough       ☐1
    aid, so that when they get home they are not     wanted more  ☐2
    quite sure how to make the best use of it.  At   n.a.         ☐3
    the time when you were given your NHS hearing
    aid, did you feel that you were given enough
    advice and guidance on how to use your aid, or
    would you have liked to have had more?

9.  What were the main problems you had in getting    no problems  ☐1
    used to your NHS aid once you got home?           problems     ☐2

    _____(open ended)_         yes   no
    _____      A   ☐1    ☐2
    _____      B   ☐1    ☐2
    _____      C   ☐1    ☐2

10a.  Have you ever had a hearing aid from a commercial
      hearing aid dealer?                            yes   ☐1
                                                     no    ☐2

10b. If yes, I'd like to talk now about your commercial
     aid.  How often do you wear your commercial aid?     always      ☐1

                                                          often       ☐2

                                                          sometimes   ☐3

                                                          rarely      ☐4

                                                          never       ☐5


10c. How did the commercial and NHS service compare?  (PROMPT)

     _____ (open ended)   NHS better     ☐1

     _____                commercial     ☐2
                                                       better

     _____                no difference  ☐3

     _____                other          ☐4


10d. How many commercial aids have you ever had?
                                                                      ☐1
     (IF MORE THAN FOUR, CODE 4)
                                                                      ☐2

                                                                      ☐3

                                                                      ☐4


10e. Do you wear two hearing aids -- that is,
     one in each ear?                                      yes        ☐1

                                                           no         ☐2


11a. Can I ask you if you have ever been to see a doctor     yes      ☐1
     or specialist in private practice about your hearing
     loss?                                                   no       ☐2


11b. If yes, who paid for it?                          self           ☐1

                                                       employer        ☐2

                                                       other          ☐3

12a. Have you ever had any other help or advice from any
other persons or workers who knows about hearing loss?     yes  [1]
(PROMPT)
                                                           no   [2]
12b. If yes, who was it?

_____(open ended)__  social worker      [1]

_____  expert on deafness  [2]

_____  teacher            [3]

_____  club member        [4]

_____  deaf person        [5]

_____  other              [6]


13. Do you think your hearing loss has in any way
caused you to rely on lipreading?                          yes  [1]

                                                           no   [2]

                                                           don't
                                                           know  [3]
                                                           (d.n.)


14. Did the hearing aid clinic give you any information
about lipreading classes?                                  yes  [1]

                                                           no   [2]


15. Have you ever been to lipreading classes?              yes  [1]

                                                           no   [2]


   15a. If yes, are you attending now?                     yes  [1]

                                                           no   [2]

   15b. If yes, how long have you attended/did    up to 3 months  [1]
        you attend?
                                                  3-6 months      [2]

                                                  7-11 months     [3]

                                                  1-5 years       [4]

                                                  more than 5     [5]
                                                       years

15c.  How helpful did you/do you find the
      classes?                                    very helpful      $\boxed{1}$

                                                  quite helpful     $\boxed{2}$

                                                  not very helpful  $\boxed{3}$


15d.  How much have the classes improved
      your lipreading?                            a lot             $\boxed{1}$

                                                  a fair amount     $\boxed{2}$

                                                  a little          $\boxed{3}$

                                                  not at all        $\boxed{4}$


(ONLY ASK FOR THOSE INTERVIEWED AT RNID)


16a.  Had you ever heard of the RNID before we got
      in touch with you to come here today?              yes   $\boxed{1}$

                                                         no    $\boxed{2}$


16b.  If yes, have you gotten in touch with the          yes   $\boxed{1}$
      RNID for any reason?
                                                         no    $\boxed{2}$


17a.  Can you tell me the names of any (other) group,
      association, or organisation (however small) which
      helps people with a hearing loss?

17b.  Which ones have you ever been in touch with?

(DO NOT PROMPT)

|            | RNID | BAHOH | BDA | NDCS | City Lit. | Link | Loc. Soc. | Other |
|------------|------|-------|-----|------|-----------|------|-----------|-------|
| a. not heard of | 1 | 1 | 1 | 1 | 1 | 1 | 1 | 1 |
| b. heard of only | 2 | 2 | 2 | 2 | 2 | 2 | 2 | 2 |
| c. heard of and been in touch | 3 | 3 | 3 | 3 | 3 | 3 | 3 | 3 |

18.  People often find that they can get some help in their day-to-day lives by having technical aids in their homes, such as special fitments to the doorbell, flashing alarm clocks, etc.  What special aids have you heard of and which do you have?

| type of aid | not heard of | heard of | heard of and got |
|-------------|--------------|----------|------------------|
| television  | 1 | 2 | 3 |
| phone       | 1 | 2 | 3 |
| doorbell    | 1 | 2 | 3 |
| alarm clock | 1 | 2 | 3 |
| baby alarm  | 1 | 2 | 3 |
| other       | 1 | 2 | 3 |

19.  Does your hearing loss prevent you from using the telephone?

yes [1]

no [2]

20.  People have different ideas about what makes somebody a handicapped person.  Someone who is confined to a wheelchair is obviously handicapped, while someone who needs a walking stick may or may not be thought of as handicapped.

A person who is completely blind is handicapped, while someone who is prevented from having a driving license because of poor eyesight may or may not be thought of as handicapped.

Do you consider that having hearing loss makes you yourself a handicapped person?

yes [1]

no [2]

21a.  Do you tend to tell people that you are deaf fairly
      soon after meeting them?                      tends to        ☐1

                                                    tends not to    ☐2


21b.  Why is that so?

                        (open ended)                              yes    no

      _____      tend to      A        ☐1    ☐2

      _____                   B        ☐1    ☐2

      _____                   C        ☐1    ☐2

      _____

      _____      tends not    D        ☐1    ☐2

      _____      to           E        ☐1    ☐2

      _____                   F        ☐1    ☐2


22.   Are you married, widowed, single,               married        ☐1
      separated, or divorced? (If not married,
      skip to Q. 25.)                                 widowed        ☐2

                                                      single         ☐3

                                                      separated      ☐4

                                                      divorced       ☐5


23.   If married, is this your first marriage?          yes        ☐1

                                                        no         ☐2


24.   Has your husband/wife ever been recommended
      to wear a hearing aid?                            yes        ☐1

                                                        no         ☐2

Now I'd like to talk about your schooling.

25. Did you pass any recognised examinations     No/none     ⌐0⌐

     as part of your education or training?     CSE     ⌐1⌐

     Did you complete an apprenticeship?

     (ONLY RING CODE IS ANSWER GIVEN     GCE "O" level/Ordinary

     CORRESPONDS EXACTLY TO THE WORDING ON     National Certificate/

     THE PRECODES. IF IT DOES NOT, RING     Ordinary National     ⌐2⌐

     "OTHER" AND RECORD DETAILS USING WORDS,               Diploma

     NOT INITIALS. NO MULTICODES POSSIBLE.     RSA/City & Guilds/

     IF MORE THAN ONE APPLIES, RING THE     Ordinary School Certi-

     HIGHEST CODE.)     ficate/Matriculation

                                     Full Industrial     ⌐3⌐

                                     Apprenticeship

                                     GCE "A" level/SRN/

                                     Higher School

                                     Certificate     ⌐4⌐

                                     Teachers Training     ⌐5⌐

                                     Certificate

                                     Higher National Certi-

                                     ficate

                                     Higher National Diploma     ⌐6⌐

                                     University Degree     ⌐7⌐

                                     Other

                                     Other (SPECIFY)

26. Now I'd like to know something     Yes, employed (including sick     ⌐1⌐

     about your employment. Are you     who are still on full pay)

     at present working for pay?     Unemployed but actively seeking     ⌐2⌐

     (IF NO, PROBE) Are you a     employment (registered at Labour

     housewife, student, retired,     Exchange)

     sick, or unemployed?     Temporarily sick (not receiving

     (CODE ANYONE WHO DOES A PAID     pay at present but has job to     ⌐3⌐

     JOB FOR MORE THAN 8 HOURS PER     return to)

     WEEK AS EMPLOYED, EVEN IF A     Retired     ⌐4⌐

     HOUSEWIFE, RETIRED, OR SELF-     Housewife (full-time)     ⌐5⌐

     EMPLOYED)     Student     ⌐6⌐

                                       Permanently sick, disabled, or

                                     unemployed not seeking     ⌐7⌐

                                     employment

                                     Other (SPECIFY)     ⌐8⌐

(IF CODED 2 or 4 PLEASE ASK Q. 27 ABOUT RESPONDANT'S LAST MAIN JOB AND
USE THE PAST TENSE. MAKE SURE EVERY QUESTION IS ASKED.)

(FOR THOSE WORKING ONLY, i.e. CODED 1, 2, or 3 IN PREVIOUS QUESTION)

27.  What job do you do?  What does   _____
     that actually involve?  Do you   _____
     hold any particular position, any_____
     rank or title for instance?      _____
     (IF STILL NOT VERY CLEAR PROMPT)_____
     Can you give me an idea of what you  _____
     do in an average day at work?    _____
     (WRITE DOWN AS DETAILED A        _____
     DESCRIPTION AS POSSIBLE)         _____

27a. Derived variable:  socioeconomic grade            I      [1]

                                                       II     [2]

                                                       IIIn   [3]

                                                       IIIm   [4]

                                                       IV     [5]

                                                       V      [6]

28a.  Are you self-employed or do you
      work for someone else?              self-employed    [1]

                                          employee         [2]

28b.  If self-employed, how many
      employees do you have?

|  |  |
|---|---|
| none | 1 |
| less than 10 | 2 |
| 10-24 | 3 |
| 25-49 | 4 |
| 50-99 | 5 |
| 100-500 | 6 |
| 501-1000 | 7 |

(DO NOT ASK)

29.  ASSESSMENT OF JOB SUITABILITY:-
     (including noise)                        0 1 2 3 4 5 6
     (TO BE COMPLETED POST HOC
     COMMENTS)

(Q. 30-32 ARE INCLUDED FOR SEG CODING ONLY.  ASK OF ALL WOMEN WHO ARE
MARRIED/SEPARATED/WIDOWED.)

30.  I would like to know something
     about your husband's employment.   yes, employed (including sick     1
     Is he at present working for pay?  who is still on (full) pay)
     (IF WIDOWED ASK IN PAST TENSE)     unemployed but actively
                                        seeking employment (registered    2
                                        at Labour Exchange)

                                        temporarily sick (not receiving
                                        pay at present but has job to      3
                                        return to)

                                        retired                            4

     (IF CODED 2 OR 4 ABOVE, PLEASE ASK ABOUT HUSBAND'S LAST MAIN JOB AND
     USE PAST TENSE.)

31.  What job does he do?  What does that actually    _____
     involve?  Does he hold any particular position,  _____
     any rank or title for instance?  (IF STILL NOT   _____
     VERY CLEAR PROMPT)  Can you give me an idea of    _____
     what he does in an average day at work?           _____
     (WRITE DOWN AS DETAILED A DESCRIPTION AS          _____
     POSSIBLE)
                                                       _____
                                                       (CODE SEG AT Q. 27)


32a. Is he self-employed or does he work for
     someone else?                                     self-employed    1

                                                       employee         2

32b. If self-employed, how many
     employees does he have?                           none             1

                                                       less than 10     2

                                                       10-24            3

                                                       25-49            4

                                                       50-99            5

                                                       100-500          6

                                                       501-1000         7


     (FOR THOSE NOT WORKING ADMINISTER DSSI AND TURN TO Q. 44.)


     (FOR THOSE WORKING ONLY)

     Now let's talk about your work.
                                                          thought  actually
33a. Has your deafness ever made you think                 of it    changed
     of giving up your job, or has it        Yes             1         3
     actually made you change your job
     recently?                               No              2         4


33b. If actually changed job, did this                           yes  1
     change of job, due to your deafness,
     mean less responsibility for you?                            no  2

                                                                 d.k. 3

34. Have you yourself made any real attempt to alter        yes   ☐1
    or rearrange your present job so that you can
    manage better?                                          no    ☐2

                                                            n.a.  ☐3


35. Have the people you work with made any                  yes   ☐1
    real attempt to alter or rearrange your
    job so that you can manage better?                      no    ☐2

                                                            n.a.  ☐3


36. All in all, how much does your hearing
    loss affect you at work?                  a lot                 ☐1

                                              from time to time     ☐2

                                              almost never          ☐3

                                              not at all            ☐4


37. Do you think you could do a more
    demanding job, would you prefer a         could do more demanding   ☐1
    less demanding job, or do you think
    that your present job is about right      would prefer less         ☐2
    for your abilities?                       demanding

                                              present job about right   ☐3


    (FOR SELF-EMPLOYED SKIP TO Q. 41)


38. And how likely do you think it is         very likely      ☐1
    that you will be promoted in the
    next five years?  Is it ...?              quite likely     ☐2
    (ONLY CODE N.A. IF VOLUNTEERED)
                                              rather unlikely  ☐3

                                              very unlikely    ☐4

                                              n.a.             ☐5

39a. People say that no one understands
     what it's like to be hard of hearing.              employer    colleagues
     Do you think that your present        yes              1            1
     employer shows any understanding of   no               2            2
     what it's like to be hard of hearing  unaware          3            3
     or not?
                                           n.a.             4            4


39b. And what of your colleagues?


40.  If your hearing gets any worse, do you                      yes      1
     think you will get any help from your
     employer or not?                                            no       2

                                                                 d.k.     3

                                                                 n.a.     4


41.  Do you expect that you will stay in          stay/not change        1
     your present job for the next five
     years or do you intend to try to             change because
     change jobs?                                 unhappy                 2
     Changing jobs means changing
     employers.                                   change because          3
                                                  career plans
     If change intended, is that
     because you are unhappy with                 n.a.                    4
     something about your present job
     or would it be part of your career
     plans?
     (ONLY CODE N.A. IF VOLUNTEERED)


     (SHOW CARD B)
42.  Here is a scale. We want to use it       ENTER BOX NO.
     now to measure how happy or unhappy      (IF NECESSARY YOU MAY PROMPT
     you are with your job. 10 represents     WITH THIS VERTICAL SCALE "5
     very happy and 0 represents very         is exactly between very happy
     unhappy. Which number on the scale       and very unhappy" DO NOT
     comes closest to how happy or unhappy    USE ANY PROMPTS OTHER THAN
     you are with your job?                    THIS OR RE-READING THE
     (TAKE BACK CARD B)                        QUESTION.)

43. In general terms, from your experience
    would you say that most people who               very difficult    ☐1
    become deaf have a very difficult/quite         quite difficult    ☐2
    difficult/fairly easy task in ad-
    justing themselves to their work                 fairly easy      ☐3
    (including housework?)

(COFFEE BREAK AND PSYCHIATRIC SCREENING DEVICE (SAD))

Now I'd like to talk about friendship

44. Some people feel that they have <u>a lot</u>    more than most people    ☐1
    of friends and some people feel that
    they don't. What would you say of              as many as most people   ☐2
    yourself? That you have ...                    fewer than most people   ☐3
                                                    none                     ☐4

45. Some people find it more difficult                   very easy          ☐1
    than others to make new friends.
    Generally speaking do you find                      fairly easy         ☐2
    making friends very easy, fairly                   quite difficult      ☐3
    easy, quite difficult, or very
    difficult?                                          very difficult      ☐4

46. Some people like chatting or passing
    the time of day with casual friends,                 enjoys             ☐1
    neighbours, workmates and so on, and               doesn't enjoy        ☐2
    some people don't. In general do you
    enjoy this or not?

47a.   We all have different ideas about what
       being lonely is.  It may have very
       little to do with the number of friends        yes    [1]
       you have or the number of people you            no     [2]
       know.  Would you describe yourself as
       a lonely person?


       (ASK EITHER B OR C.)


47b.   If no, even though you're not a lonely          often        [1]
       person, most people do have lonely patches      sometimes    [2]
       from time to time.  Would you say that you
       feel that way often, sometimes, rarely or       rarely       [3]
       never?                                          never        [4]


47c.   If yes, how often would you say that            always       [1]
       you feel that way?  Always, often,              often        [2]
       sometimes, rarely or never?
                                                       sometimes    [3]
                                                       rarely       [4]
                                                       never        [5]


48a.   Do you think that those nearest to you          yes    [1]
       understand what it is like to lose one's        no     [2]
       hearing and have to wear an aid or not?


48b.   If no, is there anyone you know who you feel    yes    [1]
       understands what it is like?                    no     [2]


49a.   To whom do you mainly turn for support          no one        [1]
       in your day-to-day life?                        spouse        [2]
                                                       family        [3]
                                                       deaf person   [4]
                                                       friend        [5]
                                                       other         [6]

49b. If supported, if it wasn't for this person who          someone    1
     would you turn to?                                        no one    2

                                                                 d.k.    3
     (SPECIFY IF SOMEONE)

_____ (open ended) _____

_____   1

_____   2

_____   3

_____   4

_____   5


50a. Do you think it would be a good thing if                     yes    1
     someone helped you to explain to your                         no    2
     family what it is like to manage with
     poor hearing?                                               n.a.    3


50b. If yes, what kind of person do you think               d.k.    1
     that should be?
     (DO NOT PROMPT)                                social worker    2

other: _____              deaf person    3

_____         other (SPECIFY)   4

_____


51a. How many other people do you know
     fairly well who have a hearing loss?            6 or more    1

                                                          4-5    2

                                                          2-3    3

                                                            1    4

                                                         none    5

51b. If none, do you think it would help you to be put
     in touch with others who have similar problems?       yes   1

                                                  no    2

                                               d.k.  3

     I expect your deafness is important in the family.
     Can we discuss it?

52. Many people say that within a family one        true    1
    member of the other may get left out of
    discussions and decision making.  Would     not true  2
    you say that was true of you or not?

    (FOR THOSE WHO HAVE EVER BEEN MARRIED)

53. How many children have you got?
    (IF MORE THAN NINE CODE 9)

54a. Can you tell me how many people live     (INTERVIEWERS CHECK)
     with you regularly in your household
     including any children.  That is, the     number in household
     people who are catered for by the
     same person as caters for you.

54b. Could you tell me the age of each person (AND IF RELEVANT ASK FOR SEX)
you have mentioned.

(FIRST ESTABLISH WHO IS THE HEAD OF THE HOUSEHOLD)

head of household     ☐1

| person number | Age | Sex M F | Relationship to head of household |
|---|---|---|---|

not head of household ☐2

1             head of household

2

3

4

5

6

7

8

9

responsible    ☐1

(scale)    ☐2

☐3

☐4

☐5

dependent

| | A | B | C | D |
|---|---|---|---|---|

(RING PERSON NUMBER OF RESPONDANT
INTERVIEWED)

A   ☐1 ☐2 ☐3 ☐4 ☐5
B   ☐1 ☐2 ☐3 ☐4 ☐5
C   ☐1 ☐2 ☐3 ☐4 ☐5
D   ☐1 ☐2 ☐3 ☐4 ☐5

(FOR MARRIED PEOPLE ONLY.  FOR ALL OTHERS SKIP TO Q. 60 OR 62.)

55. How much time do you think you spend doing
things together with your wife/husband?

quite a lot     ☐1

a moderate amount   ☐2

a little time     ☐3

56. Generally speaking, do you tell your
wife/husband about what went on
during your day?

always     ☐1

usually     ☐2

about half the time   ☐3

seldom     ☐4

never     ☐5

57.  What about your wife/husband?  Does        always                    ☐1
     she/he usually tell you what went on
     during her/his day?                        usually                   ☐2

                                                about half the time       ☐3

                                                seldom                    ☐4

                                                never                     ☐5


58.  Every husband and wife tend to fall out from time to time.  For
     example, if I was to ask you if you and your husband/wife tend to
     have rows about irritating personal habits I am sure you would be
     quite likely to say "yes, we do tend to have rows about that."
     I'm going to read you out a list of things that we have found some
     people disagree about, and I want you to say whether generally
     speaking they cause you and your husband/wife to have rows or not.

                                                        yes      no     n.a.

     A. Deciding whether to see friends together        ☐1     ☐2     ☐3

     B. Getting on with your neighbours                 ☐1     ☐2     ☐3

     C. Your being overtired                            ☐1     ☐2     ☐3

     D. Getting on with your in-laws                    ☐1     ☐2     ☐3

     E. Disciplining the children                       ☐1     ☐2     ☐3

     F. Your husband/wife not listening to what you're  ☐1     ☐2     ☐3
        saying

     G. Going out together                              ☐1     ☐2     ☐3

     H. One of you not showing enough affection         ☐1     ☐2     ☐3

     I. About nothing in particular                     ☐1     ☐2     ☐3

     J. About situations arising from your deafness     ☐1     ☐2     ☐3


59.  All in all, how do you think your hearing
     impairment has affected your marriage...?       a lot              ☐1

                                                     from time to time  ☐2

                                                     almost never       ☐3

                                                     not at all         ☐4

(FOR THOSE WITH CHILDREN.  FOR THOSE WITH NO CHILDREN SKIP TO Q. 62)

60. How much time would you say you spend
    doing things with your child(ren)...?          quite a lot        [1]

                                                    moderate amount    [2]

                                                    relatively little  [3]

61. Do you tend to enjoy the company of your             tends to   [1]
    children's friends or not?                          tends not   [2]

(FOR EVERYONE)

62. I'd like to ask you (again) how much
    you think your hearing impairment has       a lot              [1]
    affected your family life ...?
                                                from time to time  [2]

                                                almost never       [3]

                                                not at all         [4]

                                                n.a.               [5]

(HEALTH)

Now I would like to ask you a few questions about your health.

63. Do you, yourself, have any long standing       no trouble        [1]
    physical disability or health trouble
    other than your hearing impairment?          yes not limited   [2]
    If yes, does it keep you from doing
    things you might like to do?                 yes limits me     [3]

(SHOW CARD C)

|  |  | not at<br>all | a<br>little | quite<br>a lot | a<br>great<br>deal | d.k./<br>n.a. |
|---|---|---|---|---|---|---|
| 64a. | To what extent, if any, do you have trouble <u>getting to sleep</u> <u>at night</u> nowadays? | 1 | 2 | 3 | 4 | 9 |
| 64b. | And to what extent, if any, do you have trouble <u>staying asleep</u>? | 1 | 2 | 3 | 4 | 9 |

(TAKE BACK CARD C)

65. In general, do you have enough energy
to do all the things that you would
like to do?

yes   1

no   2

(SHOW CARD D)

66. All things considered, how satisfied or
dissatisfied are you overall with <u>your</u>
present state of health?
(TAKE BACK CARD D)

(ENTER BOX NUMBER)

67. How good would you rate your eyesight
(with glasses on if wears them)
Excellent, fairly good, not very good
or poor?

excellent   1

fairly good   2

not very good   3

poor   4

68. Most people these days have something they worry about, sometimes big things, sometimes quite small things. To what extent, during the past few weeks have you worried... (CODE: ENTER BOX CODES BELOW)

(SHOW CARD E)

a. about not having enough money for day-to-day living

b. about financial debts such as HP, mortgage, etc.

c. about relations with neighbours

d. about your health

e. about your family

f. about how things are going at work/your husband's work

g. about Britain's future

h. about growing old

i. that you might have a nervous breakdown

69. And how much do you worry about your deafness?
In general, how much would you say you worry these days?

(TAKE BACK CARD E)

70. Have you ever consulted a doctor or anyone else to seek help about a nervous problem for yourself?
If yes, was that once or more than once?

no                          1

yes--once                   2

yes--more than once         3

71a. Generally speaking, would you say that most people can be trusted or that you can't be too careful in dealing with people?

most people can be trusted          1

can't be too careful                2

71b. Would you say that most of the time people      try to be helpful   ☐1
     try to be helpful, or that they are mostly     look out for    ☐2
     just looking out for themselves?      themselves

71c. Do you think that most people would try      take advantage   ☐1
     to take advantage of you if they got the
     chance or would they try to be fair?      try to be fair    ☐2

72. Do you think you have had a fair opportunity    fair opportunity   ☐1
     to make the most of yourself in life, or
     have you been held back in some ways?      held back      ☐2

(SHOW CARD D.  CODE 99 FOR "DON'T KNOW.")

73a. All things considered, how satisfied or dissatisfied
     are you overall with your life as a whole these days?      ☐☐

73b. And where would you put yourself as you were
     five years ago?      ☐☐

73c. And where do you expect you will be in five
     years time?      ☐☐

(TAKE BACK CARD D.)

74. We've been talking a lot about the problems of losing your hearing.
     Now let's look at it from the other side. Has loss of hearing led
     to any actual gains in your life as a whole?

_____ (open ended)      no      ☐1

_____      yes   A   ☐2

_____      yes   B   ☐3

_____      yes   C   ☐4

_____      yes   C   ☐5

(THANK RESPONDENT AND DEAL WITH EXPENSES.)

TIME COMPLETED    ☐

(PLEASE COMPLETE INTERVIEWER'S ASSESSMENT.)

Appendix A

Interviewer's Assessment


1. Emotional state (5-point scale)
    5 = very composed
    1 = very upset                         ☐


2. Co-operation
    5 = very co-operative
    1 = very unco-operative        ☐


3. Interference of hearing impairment
   with interview
    5 = very good communication
    1 = very poor communication   ☐


4. Reasons for incomplete interview:


    a.  Audiogram

    b.  Speech Discrimination

    c.  Questionnaire

    d.  SSI


5. Any other comments:

# *Second Study: Self-Completion Questionnaire*

We would like you to answer some questions about yourself.

Most of the questions can be answered by simply ticking one of the boxes like this: ☑ . In some questions, more than one box can be ticked. In a few questions, a number, such as your date of birth, is asked for while in others a written description or explanation is required.

Please read each question carefully before you answer it. Please ask the interviewer should you have any queries.

Thank you.

Name _____     SEX:     male ☐ 1
                                           female ☐ 2

Date of Birth ___ ___ ___          Age now: ☐☐
              day month year

**Occupation _____

**Husband/wife's occupation _____

  ** if not working, please give last occupation

1. Are you

                                        married? ☐ 1

                                         single? ☐ 2

                    widowed/separated/divorced? ☐ 3

2. How many people live with you?

              number of people aged 16 and over ____
                   (do not include yourself)

              number of people under 16         ____

                        none, I live alone      ☐ 3

195

3. How old were you when you first noticed that you had
   difficulty in hearing?                              _____ years old

4. And how much time do you think passed between your
   noticing that you had difficulty in hearing and going
   to see a doctor about it?                           _____ years

5. Was your hearing loss          sudden (over days)?        ☐ 1
                                  gradual (over months)?     ☐ 2
                               very gradual (over years)?    ☐ 3

6. Is your hearing          staying about the same?          ☐ 1
                                    getting worse?           ☐ 2
                                    getting better?          ☐ 3
                       varying from one time to another?     ☐ 4
                                       don't know            ☐ 5

7. Do you know what caused your hearing loss?
                               It was caused by illness       ☐ 1
                               (please specify _____
                               _____)
                    I was born deaf or with poor hearing      ☐ 2
                    It was caused by an accident/injury        ☐ 3
                    (please specify _____
                    _____)
                               It was caused by noise          ☐ 4
                       It was caused by something else         ☐ 5
                       (please specify _____
                       _____)
                                       I don't know            ☐ 6

8. Do you suffer from any other complaints?        yes        ☐ 1
   If yes, what? _____           no        ☐ 2

9. Are you under the care of the doctor or the hospital at the moment?

   If yes, what for? _____          yes  ☐ 1

                                                       no   ☐ 2

10. How old were you when you first had a hearing aid?

                                             _____ years old

11. If you use a hearing aid, do you use it
    (please tick the boxes that apply to you)

    |  | does not apply | never | some-times | most of the time |
    |---|---|---|---|---|
    | at work? | ☐ 1 | ☐ 2 | ☐ 3 | ☐ 4 |
    | at home? | | ☐ 1 | ☐ 2 | ☐ 3 |
    | in the street? | | ☐ 1 | ☐ 2 | ☐ 3 |
    | when you are alone? | | ☐ 1 | ☐ 2 | ☐ 3 |

12. How many hours a day do you use your aid?

                     approximately _____ hours a day

13. At present, are you
    |  |  |
    |---|---|
    | employed? | ☐ 1 |
    | self-employed? | ☐ 2 |
    | retired? | ☐ 3 |
    | not working but seeking employment? | ☐ 4 |
    | not working and not seeking employment? | ☐ 5 |
    | other? (please specify _____) | ☐ 6 |

Answer only if you are working at present

14. What is your job? _____

15. Please give a brief description of what your job entails. _____

_____

_____

16. Do you work full-time or part-time?          full-time    ☐ 1

                                                 part-time    ☐ 2

17. Do you think your hearing loss has ever affected

                                    your work?    yes    ☐ 1

                                                 no     ☐ 2

                        your job prospects?       yes    ☐ 1

                                                 no     ☐ 2

18. If your hearing loss has ever affected either your work and/or your
    job prospects, did/does it do so by making it (please tick the boxes
    that apply to you)

    Work:                         difficult to use the telephone?    ☐ 1

        difficult to cope with the general public e.g. customers?    ☐ 1

                difficult to deal with the people you work with?     ☐ 1

                How? _____

                difficult to deal with your employer/supervisor?    ☐ 1

                    more difficult to do your job satisfactorily?    ☐ 1

    necessary to make alterations in your job in order to cope?      ☐ 1

                        difficult to make friends at work?           ☐ 1

                    you feel left out of things at work?             ☐ 1

            people you work with have less respect for you?          ☐ 1

    Job prospects:                the cause of loss of promotion?    ☐ 1

                                   the cause of loss of job?         ☐ 1

                          the cause of loss of responsibility?       ☐ 1

                the cause of demotion to a lower paid job?           ☐ 1

Answer only if you are not working at present

19. Have you ever worked?                          yes    ☐ 1
                                                   no     ☐ 2

Answer only if you have NEVER worked:

20. Has your hearing loss ever had anything to do with
    your not working?                                    yes    ☐ 1

                                                          no     ☐ 2

If yes, how? _____

_____

_____

_____


Answer only if you have EVER worked:

21. How old were you when you stopped work?      _____  years old


22. Did your hearing loss have anything to do with your    yes    ☐ 1
    stopping work?                                         no     ☐ 2

23. What was your last job?    _____

24. Please give a brief description of what your last job entailed.

    _____

    _____

    _____


25. Did you work full-time or part-time in your last job?

                                               full-time   ☐ 1

                                               part-time   ☐ 2


26. Do you think your hearing loss ever affected

                                  your work? yes    ☐ 1

                                          no        ☐ 2

                       your job prospects? yes      ☐ 1

                                          no        ☐ 2

27. If your hearing loss did affect either your work and/or your
    job prospects, did it do so by making it (please tick the
    boxes that apply to you)

Work:                                  difficult to use the telephone?      ☐ 1

    difficult to cope with the general public e.g. customers etc.?          ☐ 1

                     difficult to deal with the people you work with?       ☐ 1

        How?    _____

                     difficult to deal with your employer/supervisor?      ☐ 1

        How?    _____

                     more difficult to do your job satisfactorily?         ☐ 1

    necessary to make alterations in your job in order to cope?             ☐ 1

                          difficult to make friends at work?                ☐ 1

                          you feel left out of things at work?              ☐ 1

            people you work with have less respect for you?                 ☐ 1


Job prospects:                         the cause of loss of promotion?      ☐ 1

                               the cause of loss of job?                    ☐ 1

                     the cause of loss of responsibility?                   ☐ 1

            the cause of demotion to a lower paid job?                      ☐ 1


28. How has your hearing loss affected your relationship with
    your family and friends?   _____

    _____

    _____

    _____


29. Any other comments you may like to add about living with a
    hearing loss:   _____

    _____

    _____

30. Would you be prepared to be interviewed again, possibly in
    your own home?                                    yes    ☐ 1

                                                       no     ☐ 2


Now please check that you have answered all the questions.

Thank you for completing the questionnaire.

# References

Abel, R. A. (1976). An investigation into some aspects of visual handicap. *Statistical Research Report Series 14*. Department of Health and Social Security, London.

Ashley, J. (1973). "Journey into Silence." Bodley Head, London.

Ballantyne, J. (1977). "Deafness." Churchill, London.

Barcham, L. J. and Stephens, S. D. G. (1980). The use of an open-ended problems questionnaire in auditory rehabilitation. *British Journal of Audiology* **14,** 49–58.

Barker, R. G., Wright, B. A., Meyerson, L., and Gonick, M. R. (1953). "Adjustment to physical handicap and illness: A survey of the social psychology of physique and disability" (Bulletin 55). Social Science Research Council, New York.

Barr, T. (1886). Enquiry into the effects of loud sounds upon the hearing of boiler makers and others who work in noisy surroundings. *Proceedings of the Philosophical Society of Glasgow* **17,** 223–239.

Bedford, A., and Foulds, G. A. (1978). "The Personal Distress Inventory and Scales." National Foundation for Educational Research, Windsor, Berkshire.

Beethoven, L. van. (1802). Heiligenstadt Document. *In* "Letters of Beethoven" (E. Anderson, ed.). Macmillan, London.

Bergman, M., Blumenfeld, V. G., Cascardo, D., Dash, B., Levitt, H., and Margulies, M. K. (1976). Age-related decrement in hearing for speech. *Journal of Gerontology* **31,** 533–538.

Bernstein, B. (1971). "Class, codes and control," Vol. I. Routledge and Kegan Paul, London.

Bird, E., and Trevains, S. (1978). "The Study of the Communication Patterns and Problems of Hearing Impaired People at Work." Report submitted to the Department of Health and Social Security, London.

Boothroyd, A. (1968). Developments in speech audiometry. *Sound* **2,** 3–20.

Bradburn, N. M. (1969). "The structure of Psychological Wellbeing." Aldine, Chicago.

Brattgard, S. O. (1974). Social and psychological aspects of the situation of the disabled. *In* "The Handicapped Person in the Community" (D. M. Boswell and J. M. Wingrove, eds.). Tavistock/Open University Press, London.

Brooks, D. N. (1981). Use of postaural aids by National Health Service patients. *British Journal of Audiology* **15,** 79–86.

Bunting, C. (1981). "Public Attitudes to Deafness." Office of Population Censuses and Surveys, Her Majesty's Stationary Office, London.

Campbell, A., Converse, P. E., and Rodger, W. L. (1976). "The Quality of American Life." Sage Foundation, New York.

Carpenter, J. O. (1974). Changing roles and disagreement in families with disabled husbands. *Archives of Physical Medicine and Rehabilitation* **55**, 272–274.

Cattell, R. B., Eber, H. W., and Tatsuoka, M. M. (1970)."Handbook for the Sixteen Personality Factor Questionnaire" (16PF). National Foundation for Educational Research, Windsor, Berkshire.

Chaiklin, J. B., and Ventry, I. M. (1963). Functional hearing loss. *In* "Modern Developments in Audiology" (J. Jerger, ed.). Academic Press, New York.

Cogswell, B. E. (1976). Conceptual model of family as a group: family response to disability. *In* "The Sociology of Physical Disability and Rehabilitation" (G. L. Albrecht, ed.). University of Pittsburgh Press.

Comer, R. J., and Piliavin, J. A. (1972). The effects of physical deviance upon face-to-face interaction: The other side. *Journal of Personality and Social Psychology* **23**, 33–39.

Conrad, R. (1977). The reading ability of deaf school leavers. *British Journal of Educational Psychology* **47**, 138–148.

Conrad, R. (1979). "The Deaf School Child: Language and Cognitive Function." Harper and Row, London.

Cooper, A. F. (1976). Deafness and psychiatric illness. *British Journal of Psychiatry* **129**, 216–226.

Cooper, A. F., Curry, A. R., Kay, D. W. K., Garside, R. F., and Roth, M. (1974). Hearing loss in paranoid and affective psychoses of the elderly. *Lancet* **2**, 851–854.

Crisp, A. H., Gaynor Jones, M., and Slater, P. (1978a). The Middlesex Hospital Questionnaire: A validity study. *British Journal of Medical Psychology* **51**, 269–280.

Crisp, A. H., Ralph, P. C., McGuiness, B., and Harris, G. (1978b). Psychoneurotic profiles in the adult population. *British Journal of Medical Psychology* **51**, 293–301.

Crown, S., and Crisp, A. H. (1979). "Crown-Crisp Experiental Index." (Formerly the Middlesex Hospital Questionnaire.) Hodder and Stoughton Educational, Sevenoaks, Kent.

Czubalski, K., Bochenek, W., and Zawisza, E. (1976). Psychological stress and personality in Ménière's disorder. *Journal of Psychosomatic Research* **20**, 187–191.

Davis, A. C. (1983). Hearing disorders in the population: First phase findings of the MRC National Study of Hearing. *In* "Hearing Science and Hearing Disorders" (M. E. Lutman and M. P. Haggard, eds.). Academic Press, London.

Davis, A. C., and Thornton, A. R. D. (1983). "Characteristics of the Adult Population in Great Britain with Severe Hearing Impairment." Proceedings of the IVth British Conference on Audiology, London.

Denmark, J. C. (1969). Management of severe deafness in adults; The psychiatrist's contribution. *Proceedings of the Royal Society of Medicine* **62**, 965–967.

Denmark, J. C. (1973). The education of deaf children. *Hearing* **28**, 3–12.

Denmark, J. C. (1976). The psycho-social implications of deafness. *Modern Perspectives in Psychiatry* **7**, 188–205.

Denmark, J. C., Rodda, M., Abel, R. A., Skelton, U., Eldridge, R. W., Warren, F., and Gordon, A. (1979). A word in deaf ears: A study of communication and behaviour in a sample of 75 deaf adolescents. Royal National Institute for the Deaf, London.

DES (1963). Health and the school child, 1962 and 1963. *Report of the Chief Medical Officer of the Department of Education and Science*. Her Majesty's Stationery Office, London.

DHSS (1973). "Deafness: Report of a departmental enquiry into the promotion of research." Department of Health and Social Security, Her Majesty's Stationery Office, London.

Dongen Garrad, J. van (1978). Personal communication.

D'Souza, M. F., Irwig, L. M., Trevelyan, H. T., Swan, A. V., Shannon, D., Tuckmann, E., and Woodall, J. T. (1975). Deafness in middle age—how big is the problem? *Journal of the Royal College of General Practitioners* **25**, 472–478.

Duckworth, D. (1983). "The classification and measurement of disablement," DHSS Social Research Branch Report No. 10. Her Majesty's Stationary Office, London.

Eastwood, M. R. (1971). Screening for psychiatric disorder. *Psychological Medicine* **1**, 197–208.

Eastwood, M. R., and Trevelyan, M. H. (1972). Relationship between physical and psychiatric disorder. *Psychological Medicine* **2**, 363–372.

Ewertsen, H. W., and Birk Nielsen, H. (1973). Social Hearing Handicap Index. *Audiology* **12**, 180–187.

Eysenck, H. J., and Eysenck, S. B. G. (1975). "Manual of the Eysenck Personality Questionnaire." National Foundation for Educational Research, Windsor, Berkshire.

Fillmore, C. J., Kempler, D., and Wang, W. S. Y. (eds.) (1979). "Individual Differences in Language Ability and Language Behaviour." Academic Press, New York.

Fink, S. L., Skipper, Jr., J. K., and Hallenbeck, P. N. (1968). Physical disability and problems in marriage. *Journal of Marriage and the Family* **30**, 64–73.

Finlay-Jones, R. A., and Burvill, P. W. (1977). The prevalence of minor psychiatric disturbance in the community. *Psychological Medicine* **7**, 475–489.

Foulds, G. A., and Bedford, A. (1975) Hierarchy of classes of personal illness. *Psychological Medicine* **5**, 181–192.

Foulds, G. A., and Hope, K. (1968). "Manual of the Symptom-Sign-Inventory (SSI). University of London Press.

Frisina, R. (ed.) (1976). "A Bicentennial Monograph on Hearing Impairment: Trends in the USA." Alexander Graham Bell Association for the Deaf Inc., New York.

Furth, H. G. (1966). "Thinking Without Language." The Free Press, New York.

Garrad, J. (1975). A controlled epidemiological study of psychological disturbance among disabled adults living in the community. *British Journal of Preventive and Social Medicine* **29**, 61.

Gildston, H., and Gildston, P. (1972). Personality changes associated with surgically corrected hypoacusis. *Audiology* **11**, 354–367.

Gilhome Herbst, K. R. (1980). "Deaf and Lonely." Royal National Institute for the Deaf, London. (Unpublished typescript.)

Gilhome Herbst, K. R., and Humphrey, C. M. (1980). Hearing impairment and mental state in the elderly living at home. *British Medical Journal* **281**, 903–905.

Gilhome Herbst, K. R., and Humphrey, C. M. (1981). The prevalence of hearing impairment in the elderly living at home. *Journal of the Royal College of General Practitioners* **31**, 155–160.

Glorig, A., Wheeler, D., Quiggle, R., Grings, W., and Summerfield, A. (1957). "1954 Wisconsin State Fair Hearing Survey." American Academy of Ophthalmology and Otolaryngology, Rochester, Minnesota.

Goffman, E. (1963). "Stigma: Notes on the Management of a Spoiled Identity." Prentice Hall, New Jersey.

Goldberg, D. P. (1972). The detection of psychiatric illness by questionnaire. *Maudsley Monographs*, No. 21. Oxford University Press.

Goldberg, D. P. (1979). Personal communication.

Goldberg, D. P., Kay, C., and Thompson, L. (1976). Psychiatric morbidity in general practice and the community. *Psychological Medicine* **6**, 565–569.

Goodman, L. A. (1970). The multivariate analysis of qualitative data: Interactions among multiple classifications. *Journal of the American Statistical Association* **65**, 226–256.

Guilford, J. P., and Zimmerman, W. S. (1949). "The Guilford-Zimmerman Temperament Survey." Sheridan Supply, Beverly Hills, California.

Haggard, M. P., Gatehouse, S., and Davis, A. (1981a). The high prevalence of hearing disorders and its implications for services in the UK. *British Journal of Audiology* **15**, 241–251.

Haggard, M. P., Foster, J. R., and Iredale, F. E. (1981b). Use and benefit of postaural aids in sensory hearing loss. *Scandinavian Audiology* **10**, 45–52.

Haines, C. M. (1927). The effects of defective hearing upon the individual as a member of the social order. *Journal of Abnormal and Social Psychology* **22**, 151–156.

Harris, A. (1971). "Handicapped and Impaired in Great Britain, Part One." Her Majesty's Stationary Office, London.

Harris, M., Thomas, A. J., and Lamont, M. (1981). Use of environmental aids by adults with severe sensorineural hearing loss. *British Journal of Audiology* **15**, 101–106.

Hastorf, A., Wildfogel, J., and Cassman, T. (1979). Acknowledgement of handicap as a tactic in social interaction. *Journal of Personality and Social Psychology* **37**, 1790–1797.

Hebb, D. O., Heath, E. S., and Stuart, E. A. (1954). Experimental deafness. *Canadian Journal of Psychology* **8**, 152–156.

High, W. S., Fairbanks, G., and Glorig, A. (1964). Scale for self assessment of hearing loss. *Journal of Speech and Hearing Disorders* **29**, 215–230.

Hinchcliffe, R. (1967). Personal and family medical history in Ménière's disease. *Journal of Laryngology and Otology* **81**, 661–668.

Hinde, R. A. (1978). Interpersonal relationships—in quest of a science. *Psychological Medicine* **8**, 373–386.

Hodkinson, H. M. (1973). Mental impairment in the elderly. *Journal of the Royal College of Physicians* **7**, 305–317.

Hood, J. D., and Poole, J. P. (1971). Speech audiometry in conductive and sensorineural hearing loss. *British Journal of Audiology* **5**, 30–38.

Houston, F., and Royse, A. B. (1954). Relationship between deafness and psychiatric illness. *Journal of Mental Science* **100**, 990–993.

Humphrey, C., Gilhome Herbst, K., and Faruqi, S. (1981). Some characteristics of the hearing impaired elderly who do not present themselves for rehabilitation. *British Journal of Audiology* **15**, 25–30.

Hunt, W. M. (1944). Progressive deafness. *Laryngoscope*, **54**, 229–234.

Hutcherson, R. W., Dirks, D. D., and Morgan, D. E. (1979). Evaluation of the Speech Perception in Noise (SPIN) test. *Otolaryngology, Head and Neck Surgery* **87**, 239–245.

Hyde, M., Pattison, E., and Sherman, G. (1981). Survey of the perceived needs of hearing impaired adults in Queensland. *Australian Journal of Audiology* **3**, 5–10.

Ingalls, G. S. (1946). Some psychiatric observations on patients with hearing defect. *Occupational Therapy and Rehabilitation* **25**, 62–66.

Janis, I. L. (1969). "Stress and Frustration." Harcourt, New York.

Jeter, I. K. (1976). Unidentified hearing impairment among psychiatric patients. *American Speech and Hearing Association* **18**, 843–845.

Kalikow, D. N., Stevens, K. N., and Elliott, L. L. (1977). Development of a test of speech intelligibility in noise using sentence materials with controlled word predictability. *Journal of the Acoustical Society of America* **61**, 1337–1351.

Kapteyn, T. S. (1977). Satisfaction with fitted hearing aids. *Scandinavian Audiology* **6**, 147–156.

Kay, D. W. K., and Roth, M. (1961). Environmental and hereditary factors in the schizophrenia of old age. *Journal of Mental Science* **107**, 649–686.

Kay, D. W. K., Beamish, P., and Roth, M. (1964). Old age mental disorders in Newcastle upon Tyne Pt. II: A study of possible social and medical causes. *British Journal of Psychiatry* **110**, 668–682.

Kay, D. W. K., Cooper, A. F., Garside, R. F., and Roth, M. (1976). The differentiation of paranoid and affective psychoses by patients' premorbid characteristics. *British Journal of Psychiatry* **129**, 207–215.

Keegan, D. L., Ash, D., and Greenough, T. (1976). Adjustment to blindness. *Canadian Journal of Ophthalmology* **11**, 22–29.

Knapp, P. H. (1948). Emotional aspects of hearing loss. *Psychosomatic Medicine* **10**, 203–222.

Kraepelin, E. (1915). Der Verfolgungswahn der Schwerhöringen. *In* "Psychiatrie Auflage 8," Band IV. Barth, Leipzig.

Levine, E. S. (1960). "The Psychology of Deafness: Techniques of Appraisal for Rehabilitation." Columbia University Press, New York.

Lieth, L. von der (1972a). Experimental social deafness. *Scandinavian Audiology* **1**, 81–87.

Lieth, L. von der (1972b). Hearing Tactics. *Scandinavian Audiology* **1**, 155–160.

Lindsey, P. H., and Norman, D. A. (1972). "Human Information Processing." Academic Press, New York.

Lutman, M. E. (1983). The scientific basis for the assessment of hearing. *In* "Hearing Science and Hearing Disorders" (M. E. Lutman and M. P. Haggard, eds.). Academic Press, London.

Lutman, M. E., and Haggard, M. P., eds. (1983). "Hearing Science and Hearing Disorders." Academic Press, London.

Lysons, J. K. (1978). "Your Hearing Loss and How to Cope with it." Royal National Institute for the Deaf, London.

MacAdam, D. B., Siegerstetter, J., and Smith, M. C. A. (1981). Deafness in adults: Screening in general practice. *Journal of the Royal College of General Practitioners* **31**, 161–164.

McCartney, J. H., Maurer, J. F., and Sorenson, F. D. (1976). A comparison of the Hearing Handicap Scale and the Hearing Measurement Scale with standard audiometric measures on a geriatric population. *Journal of Auditory Research* **16**, 51–58.

McClelland, H. A., Roth, M., Neubauer, H., and Garside, R. F. (1968). Some observations on case material based on patients with some common schizophrenic symptoms. *Proceedings of the Fourth World Congress of Psychiatry*, Vol. 4, pp. 2955–2957. Excerpta Medica, London.

McCormick, B. (1979a). Review of BBC television series on lipreading. *Hearing* **34**, 126–130.

McCormick, B. (1979b). A comparison between a two dimensional and a three dimensional lipreading test. *IRCS Medical Science* **7**, 324.

McCormick, B. (1980) "Aural rehabilitation—Phase II." Department of Health and Social Security, London.

McDaniel, J. W. (1976). "Physical Disability and Human Behaviour." Pergamon Press, New York.

Mahapatra, S. B. (1974a). Psychiatric and psychosomatic illness in the deaf. *British Journal of Psychiatry* **125**, 450–451.

Mahapatra, S. B. (1974b). Deafness and mental health: psychiatric and psychosomatic illness in the deaf. *Acta Psychiatrica Scandinavica* **50**, 596–611.

Mahendru, R. K., Srivastav, R. N., and Sharma, D. (1978). Deafness and mental ill-health: A comparative study of deaf and non-deaf psychiatric patients. *Indian Journal of Psychiatry* **20**, 148–154.

Malone, J. R. L., and Hemsley, D. R. (1977). Lowered responsiveness and auditory signal detectability during depression. *Psychological Medicine* **7**, 717–722.

Malone, R. L. (1969). Expressed attitudes of aphasics. *Journal of Speech and Hearing Disorders* **34**, 146–151.

Markides, A. (1977). Rehabilitation of people with acquired deafness in adulthood. *British Journal of Audiology*, Supplement Number 1.

Markides, A., Brooks, D. N., Hart, F. G., and Stephens, S. D. G. (1979). Aural rehabilitation of hearing impaired adults. (Official Policy of the British Society of Audiology.) *British Journal of Audiology* **13**, 7–14.

Martin, M. C., Williams, V., and Lodge, J. J. (1971). An evaluation of noise excluding enclosures for audiometric purposes. *Sound* **5**, 90–93.

Menninger, K. A. (1924). The mental effects of deafness. *Psychoanalytical Review* **11**, 144–155.

Miles, A. (1979). Some psychosocial consequences of multiple sclerosis: Problems of social interaction and group identity. *British Journal of Medical Psychology* **52**, 321–331.

Mindel, E. D., and Vernon, M. (1971). "They Grow in Silence." National Association of the Deaf, Silver Springs, Maryland.

Moore, B. C. J. (1982). "An Introduction to the Psychology of Hearing." Academic Press, London.

Morgan, A. C. W. (1978). "The Analysis of Survey Data using GLIM." B.Sc. Dissertation in Statistics and Computing at the Polytechnic of North London.

MRC (1957). Medical Research Council: Report of working party for research in general practice. *Lancet* **2**, 510.

Mueller, J. H., Schuessler, K. F., and Costner, H. L. (1970). "Statistical Reasoning in Sociology." Houghton Mifflin, Boston.

Myklebust, H. R. (1964). "The Psychology of Deafness." Grune & Stratton, New York.

Nelder, J. A., and Wedderburn, R. W. M. (1972). Generalised linear models. *Journal of the Royal Statistical Society* **135**, 370–384.

Nett, E. (1960). "The relationships between audiological measures and handicap: A project of the University of Pittsburgh School of Medicine and the Office of Vocational Rehabilitation." United States Department of Health, Education and Welfare, Washington.

Nie, N. H., Hadlai Hull, C., Jenkins, J. G., Steinbrenner, K., and Bent, D. H. (1975). "Statistical Package for the Social Sciences" (SPSS). McGraw-Hill, New York.

Noble, W. G. (1969). A scale for the measurement of hearing loss and disability. PhD. thesis, University of Manchester.

Noble, W. G. (1971). "Test Manual for the Hearing Measurement Scale." Department of Psychology, University of New England, Armidale, Australia.

Noble, W. G. (1978). "Assessment of Impaired Hearing." Academic Press, New York.

Noble, W. G. (1979). The Hearing Measurement Scale as a paper[pencil form: Preliminary results. *Journal of the American Auditory Society* **5**, 95–106.

Noble, W. G. (1983). Hearing, hearing impairment and the audible world: A theoretical essay. *Audiology* **22**, 325–338.

Noble, W. G., and Atherley, G. R. C. (1970). The Hearing Measure Scale: A questionnaire for the assessment of auditory disability. *Journal of Auditory Research* **10**, 229–250.

O'Muircheartaigh, C. A., and Payne, C. (eds.). (1977). "The Analysis of Survey Data." Wiley, London.

Peterson, A. P. G., and Gross, Jr., E. E. (1972). "Handbook of Noise Measurement." General Radio, Concord, Massachusetts.

Phillips, W. C., and Rowell, H. G. (1932). "Your Hearing: How to Preserve and Aid It." Appleton, New York.

Post, F. (1966). "Persistent Persecutory States of the Elderly." Pergamon, London.

Ramsdell, D. A. (1962). The psychology of the hard-of-hearing and deafened adult. *In* "Hearing and Deafness" (H. Davis and S. R. Silverman, eds.). Holt, Rhinehart and Winston, New York.

Rawson, A. (1973). The everyday consequences of acquired deafness. *Hearing* **28**, 76–78.

Remmers, H. H., and Wright, G. N. (1960). "The Purdue Handicap Problems Inventory." Purdue University, Lafayette, Indiana.

Rosen, J. K. (1979). Psychological and social aspects of the evaluation of acquired hearing impairment. *Audiology* **18**, 238–252.

Rosen, S., Bergman, M., Plester, D., El-Mofty, A., and Satti, M. (1962). Presbyacusis study of a relatively noise free population in the Sudan. *Annals of Otology, Rhinology and Laryngology* **71**, 727–743.

Savill, S. (1975). My side of the fence. *Rehabilitation* **95**, 4–6.

Schein, J. D., and Delk, M. R. (1975). "The Deaf Population in the United States." National Association of the Deaf, Silver Spring, Maryland.

Shakespeare, R. (1975). "The Psychology of Handicap." Methuen, London.

Shepherd, M., Cooper, B., Brown, A. C., and Kalton, G. (1966). "Psychiatric Illness in General Practice." Oxford University Press.

Shontz, F. C. (1970). Physical disability and personality. *Rehabilitation Psychology* **17**, 51–69.

Skamris, N. P. (1974). Assessment of lipreading ability of deafened persons. *Scandinavian Audiology*, Supplement 4, 128–135.

SSRC (1981). "Psychological Research on the Family" (Newsletter No. 43). Social Science Research Council, London.

SSRC Survey Unit (1975a). "The Multipurpose Survey." Social Science Research Council Survey Unit, London.

SSRC Survey Unit (1975b). "The Quality of Life Survey." Social Science Research Council Survey Unit, London.

Stankov, L., and Horn, J. L. (1980). Human abilities revealed through auditory tests. *Journal of Educational Psychology* **72**, 21–44.

Stephens, S. D. G. (1973). Some personality factors influencing hearing. *In* "Disorders of Auditory Function" (W. Taylor, ed.). Academic Press, London.

Stephens, S. D. G. (1977). Hearing aid used by adults: A survey of surveys. *Clinical Otolaryngology* **2**, 385–402.

Stephens, S. D. G. (1979a). Can lipreading be taught? *Clinical Otolaryngology* **4**, 3–4.

Stephens, S. D. G. (1979b) "Does presbyacusis exist?'' Paper presented at a conference of the British Society of Audiology on "Hearing of Older People" in January, 1979, London.

Stephens, S. D. G. (1980). Evaluating the problems of the hearing impaired. *Audiology* **19**, 205–220.

Stephens, S. D. G. (1982). Personal communication.

Stevenson, J., and Dawtrey, L. (1980). A study of private hearing aid users in London. *British Journal of Audiology* **14**, 105–114.

Summerfield, A. Q. (1983). Audio-visual speech perception, lipreading, and artifical stimulation. *In* Hearing Science and Hearing Disorders (M. E. Lutman and M. P. Haggard, eds.). Academic Press, London.

Thomas, A. J. (1981a). Acquired deafness and mental health. *British Journal of Medical Psychology* **54**, 219–229.

Thomas, A. J. (1981b). The effect of severe hearing loss on personality. *IRCS Medical Science* **9**, 941–942.

Thomas, A. J., and Gilhome Herbst, K. R. (1980a). Social and psychological effects of acquired deafness for adults of employment age. *British Journal of Audiology* **14**, 76–85.

Thomas, A. J., and Gilhome Herbst, K. R. (1980b). Acquired deafness and psychological disorder. *In* "Disorders of Auditory Function" (W. Taylor and A. Markides, eds.), Vol. III. Academic Press, London.

Thomas, A. J., and Gilhome Herbst, K. R. (1981). The effect of type of hearing loss on speech discrimination ability. *IRCS Medical Science* **9**, 233–234.

Thomas, A. J., and Ring, J. (1981). A validation study of the Hearing Measurement Scale. *British Journal of Audiology* **15**, 55–60.

Thomas, A. J., and Ring, J. (1984). The relationship between social class and speech discrimination in adults with acquired hearing loss. *IRCS Medical Science* (in press).

Thomas, A. J., Lamont, M., and Harris, M. (1982). Problems encountered at work by people with severe acquired hearing loss. *British Journal of Audiology* **16**, 39–43.

Thorndike, E. L., and Lorge, I. (1944). "The Teacher's Word Book of 30,000 Words." Teachers College, Columbia University, New York.

Tonning, F. M. (1978). Evaluation of hearing aid fitting based on patients' experience from everyday listening conditions. *Scandinavian Audiology* **7**, 13–17.

Topliss, E. (1979). "Provision for the Disabled." Basil Blackwell, Oxford.

United States Department of Health, Education and Welfare (1965). Hearing levels of adults by age and sex: US 1960–1962. *National Centre for Health Statistics, Series 11, No. 11.* United States Government Printing Office, Washington.

Watts, W. J., Ballantyne, J., and Pegg, K. S. (1980). "Aural Rehabilitation: Further Investigation into the Rehabilitation of Adults with Acquired Hearing Loss." Reginald M. Phillips Research Unit, University of Sussex, Brighton.

Weider, A., Wolff, H. G., Brodman, K., Mittelman, B., and Wechsler, D. (1948). "Cornell Index." The Psychological corporation, New York.

Weir, N. F., and Stephens, S. D. G. (1976). Personality measures in ENT outpatients. *Journal of Laryngology and Otology* **90**, 553–560.

Welles, H. H. (1932). "The Measurement of Certain Aspects of Personality Among Hard-of-hearing Adults. Teachers College, Columbia University, New York.

Wilkins, L. T. (1948). "The Prevalence of Deafness in England, Scotland and Wales."
     Central Office of Information, London.
Wing, J. K., Cooper, J. E., and Sartorius, N. (1974). "The Description and Classification of
     Psychiatric Symptoms: An Instruction Manual for the PSE and CATEGO System."
     Cambridge University Press.
Wood, P. H. N. (1980). The language of disablement: Glossary relating to disease and its
     consequences. *International Rehabilitation Medicine* **2,** 86–92.
Zimbardo, P. G., and Andersen, S. M. (1981). Induced hearing deficit generates experimen-
     tal paranoia. *Science* **212,** 1529–1531.

# *Index*

## A

Age, 14–16, 53, 64, 66, 75, 93, 109
American Quality of Life Survey, 59
Attitudes to hearing impairment, 152
Audiological medicine, 5, 25
Audiological scientists, 5, 25
Auditory dysfunction
   terminology, 1, 6–7, 150–151
   schema relating to, 5–7, 154–165

## B

Bernreuter Personality Inventory, 33–35
British Association of the Hard-of-Hearing,
   26, 63
British Deaf Association, 26

## C

Central hearing impairment, 14, 46–47
City Literary Institute Centre for the Deaf,
   London, 25
Conductive hearing loss, 11–12, 17,
   72–73
Control groups, 60–61
Cornell Index, 40–41, 56
Crown-Crisp Experiential Index, 43, 56

## D

Depression, effect on speech
   discrimination, 158–159

## E

Employment, 50, 64–65, 89–90, 95, 96,
   107, 108–109, 126, 145–149,
   162–164
Environmental aids, 23–24, 136–139,
   145, 162
EPI (Eysenck Personality Inventory), 43
EPQ (Eysenck Personality Questionnaire),
   107, 120–123, 151–153
*ETA* coefficient, 36–39

## F

Family life, 50, 91–92, 132–145,
   161–162, 164, 165

## G

General Health Questionnaire, 56–58, 153
GLIM (General Linear Interactive
   Modelling), 61–63
Guilford–Zimmerman Temperament
   Survey, 42

213